NSNA Review

Psychiatric Nursing

Consulting Editor
Christine A. Grant, Ph.D., R.N., C.S.
Assistant Professor
Psychiatric and Mental Health Nursing
University of Pennsylvania
School of Nursing
Philadelphia, Pennsylvania

Reviewers
Bruce P. Mericle, M.S., R.N.
Assistant Professor
Trenton State College
School of Nursing
Trenton, New Jersey

Sterling Alean Royes, M.S.N., R.N., A.N.P.
Clinical Nurse Specialist, Psychiatry
Adjunct Faculty, School of Nursing
University of Texas at Arlington
Arlington, Texas

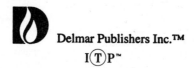

Delmar Publishers Inc.™
I(T)P™

Developed for Delmar Publishers Inc. by
  Visual Education Corporation, Princeton, New Jersey.
Publisher: David Gordon
Sponsoring Editor: Patricia Casey
Project Director: Susan J. Garver
Developmental Editor: Emilie McCardell
Production Supervisor: Amy Davis
Proofreading Management: Christine Osborne
Word Processing: Cynthia C. Feldner
Composition: Maxson Crandall, Lisa Evans-Skopas
Cover Designer: Paul C. Uhl, DESIGNASSOCIATES
Text Designer: Circa 86

For information, address
Delmar Publishers Inc.
3 Columbia Circle
Box 15015
Albany, New York 12212

Printed in the United States of America
Published simultaneously in Canada by Nelson Canada,
a division of The Thomson Corporation

10 9 8 7 6 5 4 3 2 1

Library of Congress Cataloging-in-Publication Data

Psychiatric nursing / consulting editor, Christine A. Grant; reviewers,
  Bruce P. Mericle, Sterling Alean Royes.
       p.   cm. — (NSNA review series)
    Developed for Delmar Publishers Inc. by Visual Education
  Corporation.
    ISBN 0-8273-5672-2
    1. Psychiatric nursing—Outlines, syllabi, etc.   I. Grant,
  Christine A.   II. Mericle, Bruce P.   III. Royes, Sterling Alean.
  IV. Visual Education Corporation.   V. Series.
    [DNLM: 1. Psychiatric Nursing—outlines. WY 18 P9772 1994]
  RC440.P748 1994
  610´.73´68—dc20
  DNLM/DLC
  for Library of Congress   93-37961
                                                        CIP

Notice to the Reader

The publisher, editors, advisors, and reviewers do not warrant or guarantee any of the products described herein nor have they performed any independent analysis in connection with any of the product information contained herein. The publisher, editors, advisors, and reviewers do not assume, and each expressly disclaims, any obligation to obtain and include information other than that provided to them by the manufacturer.

The reader is expressly warned to consider and adopt all safety precautions that might be indicated by the activities described herein and to avoid all potential hazards. By following the instructions contained herein, the reader willingly assumes all risks in connection with such instructions.

The publisher, editors, advisors, and reviewers make no representations or warranties of any kind, including but not limited to the warranties of fitness for particular purpose or merchantability, nor are any such representations implied with respect to the material set forth herein, and the publisher, editors, advisors, and reviewers take no responsibility with respect to such material. The publisher, editors, advisors, and reviewers shall not be liable for any special, consequential, or exemplary damages resulting, in whole or in part, from readers' use of, or reliance upon, this material.

A conscientious effort has been made to ensure that the drug information and recommended dosages in this book are accurate and in accord with accepted standards at the time of publication. However, pharmacology is a rapidly changing science, so readers are advised, before administering any drug, to check the package insert provided by the manufacturer for the recommended dose, for contraindications for administration, and for added warnings and precautions. This recommendation is especially important for new, infrequently used, or highly toxic drugs.

CPR standards are subject to frequent change due to ongoing research. The American Heart Association can verify changing CPR standards when applicable. Recommended Schedules for Immunization are also subject to frequent change. The American Academy of Pediatrics, Committee on Infectious Diseases can verify changing recommendations.

Contents

Preface

The NSNA Review Series is a multiple-volume series designed to help nursing students review course content and prepare for course tests.

Chapter elements include:

Overview—lists the main topic headings for the chapter

Nursing Highlights—gives significant nursing care concepts relevant to the chapter

Glossary—features key terms used in the chapter that are not defined within the chapter

Enhanced Outline—consists of short, concise phrases, clauses, and sentences that summarize the main topics of course content; focuses on nursing care and the nursing process; includes the following elements:
- *Client Teaching Checklists:* shaded boxes that feature important issues to discuss with clients; designed to help students prepare client education sections of nursing care plans
- *Nurse Alerts:* shaded boxes that provide information that is of critical importance to the nurse, such as danger signs or emergency measures connected with a particular condition or situation
- *Locators:* finding aids placed across the top of the page that indicate the main outline section that is being covered on a particular 2-page spread within the context of other main section heads
- *Textbook reference aids:* boxes labeled "See text pages ____," which appear in the margin next to each main head, to be used by students to list the page numbers in their textbook that cover the material presented in that section of the outline
- *Cross references:* references to other parts of the outline, which identify the relevant section of the outline by using the numbered and lettered outline levels (e.g., "same as section I,A,1,b" or "see section II,B,3")

Chapter Tests—review and reinforce chapter material through questions in a format similar to that of the National Council Licensure Examination for Registered Nurses (NCLEX-RN); answers follow the questions and contain rationales for both correct and incorrect answers

Comprehensive Test—appears at the end of the book and includes items that review material from each chapter

1

Introduction

NURSING HIGHLIGHTS

1. Diagnosis and treatment of mental illness have evolved over time and continue to evolve today; a historical perspective helps the nurse understand the context in which today's psychiatric nursing care is provided.
2. The nurse's role in the care of the mentally ill is expanding as part of current trends toward community mental health, self-help, prevention, and holistic treatment.
3. The steps in the nursing process, particularly nursing diagnosis, are the psychiatric nurse's fundamental tools in planning and providing effective care.

4. Nurse often serves as primary point of contact between the client and the mental health system.
5. Community-based programs require continuity of care between service agencies.
6. Psychiatric nurses who work in psychiatric inpatient settings provide vital teaching to help prepare client and family for client's reentry into community; this is especially important in light of the increase in short-term stays in psychiatric inpatient hospitals.
7. Psychiatric nursing skills are often applied in general nursing practice settings.

GLOSSARY

anticipatory guidance—identification of client's coping skills and, if necessary, modification of inappropriate coping skills

case-finding—method of identifying people who need treatment for mental health problems

case manager—person who assesses total needs of chronically mentally ill person and who coordinates therapeutic support service to help the individual live in the community

client advocate—individual who educates clients about their rights and responsibilities and who works to see that services clients need are made available

cognitive theory—view that emotional problems stem from faulty thinking processes

community mental health—an approach to treatment of mental illness that focuses on attempts to promote the client's ability to function within his/her community, as an alternative to institutionalization

consultation-liaison—provision of psychiatric care to medical-surgical clients in a general hospital in collaboration with medical-surgical personnel

DSM-III-R—*Diagnostic and Statistical Manual of Mental Disorders,* revised third edition, published by American Psychiatric Association in 1987; most widely used classification system for mental disorders; emphasizes specific, detailed criteria and attempts to create objective classifications that do not rely on any particular theoretic framework; fourth edition (DSM-IV) expected to be published in 1994

general systems theory—view that integrates issues of biologic and social sciences with those of physical science in examining human behavior

holism—an approach to health care that considers all the client's needs: physical, mental, social, developmental, and spiritual

ICU psychosis—also called intensive care syndrome; condition in which a client in ICU exhibits signs of depression, withdrawal, anxiety, hallucinations, delirium, or paranoia, due to sensory deprivation; may be influenced by medications, age of client, pre-ICU mental and physical condition

moral treatment—humane treatment of people who are mentally ill, practiced and promoted in the 19th century; laid foundation for modern therapeutic techniques

nursing diagnosis—a statement of a client's nursing problem, including adaptive and maladaptive health responses and contributing stressors

nursing process—an interactive, disciplined, systematic approach to planning and performing individualized nursing care; consists of cognitive and behavioral steps

primary nursing—care of a psychiatric inpatient by 1 nurse who is responsible for managing that individual's case 24 hours a day

self-help group—an approach to treating substance abuse and other disorders in which people with a similar problem meet for emotional and moral support and practical advice

ENHANCED OUTLINE

I. Historical overview of psychiatric beliefs and practices

See text pages

_____

A. Primitive beliefs and practices
   1. Magical/religious explanations: demons, witchcraft, and spirits as causes of mental illness
   2. Use of symbols and rituals for treatment

B. Ancient Greek/Roman beliefs and practices
   1. Moral explanations: continuation of view of mental illness as punishment by supernatural forces
   2. Organic explanations: introduction of definition of illness by Hippocrates and others as imbalances of body "humors"; definition of mental illness as medical problem; use of purging and bloodletting
   3. Beginnings of clinical observation and humane practices toward those with mental illness

C. Medieval beliefs and practices
   1. Return to magical/religious explanations for mental illness (e.g., demonic possession, influence of moon, witchcraft)
   2. Harsh treatments: imprisonment and banishment
   3. Establishment of first hospitals in Europe

D. Renaissance beliefs and practices
   1. Sorcery and witchcraft as explanations of mental illness
   2. Religious "treatments": exorcism, torture, death

E. 17th- and early 18th-century practices
   1. Development of asylums—emphasis on segregating the mentally ill from the public; included dungeons and physical restraints; treatment by nonphysicians
   2. Introduction of belief that mental illness stems from natural causes

F. Late 18th- and 19th-century beliefs and practices
   1. Rise of the Enlightenment: reliance on rational explanations, classification of mental disorders, observation through experiments
   2. Era of moral treatment: rejection of beatings; therapeutic treatment by physicians rather than imprisonment

3. Primitive first attempts at systematic treatment in the United States: bloodletting, purging, and other treatments now considered inhumane
4. Introduction of public mental hospitals in 19th century, leading to custodial care rather than cure
5. Rise of dynamic psychiatry: beginning of the study of influence of unconscious mental forces on person's personality and behavior

G. Foundations of contemporary beliefs and practices
   1. Rise of mental hygiene movement: humanitarian reforms in treatment of mental illness (e.g., preventive care and treatment of children)
   2. Development of new theories of causation and treatment
      a) Psychoanalytic theory (psychosexual stages of development): Freud
      b) Psychosocial stages of development: Erikson
      c) Interpersonal theory: Sullivan
      d) Stages of cognitive development: Piaget
      e) Cognitive theory: Beck, Ellis
      f) Behaviorism: Pavlov, Watson, Skinner, Wolpe
      g) General systems theory: Menninger

II. Current trends in psychiatric care

See text pages

_____

A. Treatment approaches
   1. Psychopharmacology (drug therapies)
   2. Self-help models of care
   3. Community mental health movement
   4. Holistic approach, with emphasis on relationship between mind and body
   5. Family counseling, marriage counseling, and group therapy, with emphasis on social factors (e.g., client's home life, social support)

B. Special mental health issues
   1. Focus on special populations (e.g., alcoholics, adolescents, elderly)
   2. Move toward shorter hospital stays with focus on crisis resolution rather than long-term care
   3. Research into biochemistry of the brain
   4. Closer coordination of physical and mental health services
   5. Expansion of role of paraprofessionals (informal caregivers such as trained volunteers), especially in community settings
   6. Continuing problems reaching underserved populations (e.g., poor, homeless)
   7. Lack of attention, funding, and research related to prevention of mental illness

C. Mental health and illness as a continuum
   1. Purpose: to define mental illness

2. Types
   a) Adaptive-maladaptive continuum
   b) Constructive-destructive continuum
3. Advantages: Approach gives therapist guidelines for assessing signs of mental health and mental illness in an individual; moves away from the deviance-conformity method of defining mental illness (i.e., classifying someone as mentally ill just on basis of being different from the norm).
4. Disadvantage: Because this approach takes away absolutes in determining mental illness, judgment about where behaviors fall along the continuum may vary.

D. DSM-III-R and DSM-IV
   1. Advantages: System provides easily identifiable behavioral signs of disorders, standardizes diagnoses, provides clear descriptions of diagnostic categories, permits comparison of treatment results, and permits development of standard treatment protocols.
   2. Disadvantages: Rigid classification system may overlook individual and cultural needs, may lump clients with different needs into same diagnosis, may promote rigid "cookbook" approach to treatment, and may not meet legal or other nonmedical criteria of what constitutes mental illness. (Some diagnostic definitions were due to change in DSM-IV.)
   3. Multiaxial system of evaluation: This classification system evaluates mental disorders on 5 dimensions. First 3 axes constitute official diagnosis; last 2 contain additional information for use in treatment and prognosis. (See Chapter 4, section VI, for more detailed explanation of axes.)

III. Nursing process in psychiatric care

See text pages
_____

A. Nursing assessment: includes gathering and verifying objective and subjective data about client (see Chapter 4 for more information on assessment tools)
   1. Data collected
      a) Biophysical, emotional, mental status
      b) Current and past use of drugs (prescription, over-the-counter, alcohol, illegal substances)
      c) Spiritual and cultural resources and beliefs
      d) Family/social support systems
      e) Daily activities, interaction, coping patterns
      f) Economic, environmental, and political factors
      g) Knowledge and motivation to change
      h) Knowledge of legal rights
      i) Information from family, significant others, mental health care team
   2. Data collection methods
      a) Medical, nursing, psychiatric histories
      b) Interview
      c) Observation
      d) Neurologic and physical assessment
      e) Psychologic testing

B. Nursing diagnoses
1. Focus: problems nurse can treat and how nurse can contribute to client's care
2. Components of nursing diagnoses
    a) Client's potential or actual unhealthful response
    b) Possible etiology (cause) of client's unhealthful response
    c) Data identifying client's unhealthful response
3. Categories of potential or actual health problems that may be identified in nursing diagnoses
    a) Limitations/impairments with general etiologies such as mental and emotional distress
    b) Emotional stress or crisis components of illness, pain, self-concept changes, life process changes

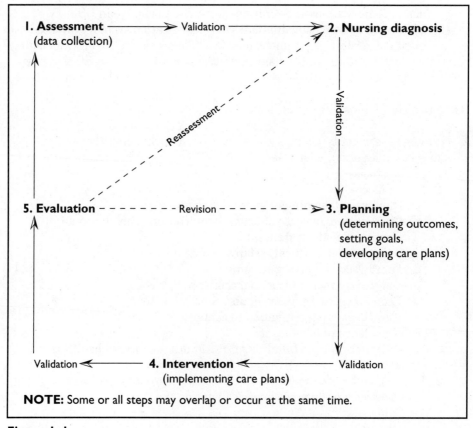

Figure 1–1
A Model for the Nursing Process

c) Emotional problems related to daily experiences such as anxiety, loss, loneliness

d) Physical symptoms (such as anorexia) occurring simultaneously with altered psychic functioning

e) Alterations in thinking, perceiving, symbolizing, communication, decision-making abilities

f) Behaviors and mental states indicating that client is dangerous to self or others or gravely disabled

4. North American Nursing Diagnosis Association (NANDA): group that has identified accepted nursing diagnoses that reflect human response patterns; provides continually updated and revised list

C. Planning: development of a nursing care plan
   1. Establishing care priorities
   2. Determining outcome criteria (short- and long-term client care goals, including those of both client and nurse)
      a) Setting realistic goals
      b) Specifying goals, including interpreting client's vague concerns into concrete goal statements
      c) Determining methods for achieving goals
   3. Using psychotherapeutic principles
   4. Indicating nurse's primary responsibilities: who will be responsible for what
   5. Continually updating and reevaluating care plan

D. Implementation of interventions: techniques
   1. Psychotherapeutic interventions for client, family, and group
   2. Health teaching
   3. Self-care activities of daily living
   4. Medications (somatic therapies)
   5. Therapeutic environment
   6. Nursing prescriptions for diet, nutrition, exercise

E. Nursing evaluation
   1. What are the outcomes (changes in client's behavior)?
   2. Which interventions were effective?
   3. Which interventions should be altered?
   4. What new interventions are necessary?
   5. Were the goals attained?

IV. Psychiatric nursing practice settings

See text pages
_____

A. Psychiatric nursing in community settings
   1. Foundations of community mental health services
      a) Provision of mental health services in the community is an outgrowth of deinstitutionalization.
      b) Community mental health care is based on the social model that emphasizes broad-based mental health services to all community members who need care.

    c) Community mental health care is based on the holistic view that people's mental health relates to their interactions with their environment (social background, support systems, family interactions).

  2. Advantages: The key advantage of community-based care is that it provides a more natural setting for the client and promotes reintegration of the client into society.

  3. Disadvantages: The disadvantages of community-based care are that it creates difficulties in supervising care, providing continuity, ensuring compliance, and ensuring access; it is easier for those needing care to "fall through the cracks"; there is an increase in homeless mentally ill who have been released from institutions.

  4. Settings: mental health centers (inpatient and outpatient), alcohol and drug treatment centers, shelters for abused women and children, day-treatment clinics, sheltered workshops for mentally retarded, crisis hotlines and clinics, homeless shelters

  5. Nurse's functions in community settings: prevention, treatment, rehabilitation

    a) Assessment, planning, implementation, and evaluation of service

    b) Crisis response services

    c) Protection and advocacy: helping client set realistic expectations for life in community and offering encouragement

    d) Peer support

    e) Family and community support

    f) Client identification: early case-finding and screening, referring clients in need of treatment

    g) Outreach services for the mentally ill who are being discharged from inpatient care: providing continuity of care (e.g., medication maintenance, home visits, social services such as finding housing and health and dental care)

    h) Teaching mental health coping skills: educating those who are at high risk for particular stressors (e.g., new mothers, adolescents whose parents are divorcing) in ways to avoid mental health problems

 B. Psychiatric nursing in psychiatric inpatient settings

  1. Nature of psychiatric inpatient facilities

    a) Increasing number of acute care facilities for short-term hospitalizations, offering variety of treatment models

    b) Long-term custodial care facilities for:

     (1) Involuntary commitments

     (2) Chronically ill who cannot function in community

     (3) Those who do not respond to treatment

      c) Skewing of inpatient population toward more difficult cases as a result of widespread deinstitutionalization

      d) Use of techniques of milieu model therapy (see Chapter 3, section III)

  2. Advantages

      a) Nurse is able to provide continuity of care to client in controlled setting.

      b) Nurse often has access to many resources (e.g., consults, peer support) to prepare a therapeutic care plan.

  3. Disadvantages

      a) The client's relative lack of control and self-determination in an institutional setting requires special attention to preserving the client's dignity and safeguarding client rights.

      b) The demands of caring for severe cases and the social structure of institutions place added stress on the nurse's personal coping mechanisms.

      c) Restrictions and regulations in an inpatient facility may cause client to be apathetic about improving condition.

  4. Nurse's function in psychiatric inpatient settings

      a) Primary nursing

      b) Client education

      c) Team member in creating care plan

      d) Crisis intervention and crisis resolution

      e) Provision of a therapeutic milieu

C. Psychiatric nursing in medical-surgical inpatient settings

  1. Background

      a) Hospitalization often presents psychologic challenges to nonpsychiatric clients and their families.

      b) Psychologic crisis situations arise among medical-surgical clients because of the following.

        (1) Fear of unknown (e.g., procedure, prognosis)

        (2) Fear of disability or death

        (3) Imminent death (care of client and family) or death of client (care of family)

        (4) Pain

        (5) Social dependency

        (6) Denial

        (7) Anxiety related to loss of autonomy, loss of control, and lack of privacy

        (8) Financial worries

        (9) Disorientation (e.g., ICU psychosis)

        (10) Deterioration of mental status

          (a) Status may be normal at admission and change during hospitalization due to disease progression, loss of mobility, or stress.

          (b) Assessment must be ongoing.

  2. Nursing implications

      a) Medical-surgical nurses must be able to identify and provide support for clients' psychologic as well as physical needs.

          b) Nurse can teach clients coping skills.
              (1) Allowing client to express feelings
              (2) Keeping client informed about all procedures
              (3) Helping client manage hospital environment
          c) Nurse may suggest need for psychiatric liaison consults.
          d) Psychiatric liaison nurses act as consultants to the medical-surgical nursing staff.
              (1) May provide consultation on specific cases
              (2) May provide in-service education on psychiatric nursing issues
              (3) May help nurses with their own psychologic needs (e.g., grieving issues for nurses treating dying clients)

1. Current research into the etiology of mental illness is focusing on which of the following as a primary factor?

   a. Urban violence
   b. Brain chemistry
   c. Alcohol dependence
   d. Parent-child relationship

2. The type of psychiatric treatment employed by groups such as Alcoholics Anonymous utilizes which model of care?

   a. Holistic
   b. Self-help
   c. Cognitive
   d. Interpersonal — STACK-Sullivan

3. One of the main advantages of the *Diagnostic and Statistical Manual of Mental Disorders* (DSM) is that it:

   a. Addresses social and cultural differences.
   b. Offers a flexible approach to diagnosis.
   c. Provides clear descriptions of diagnostic criteria.
   d. Avoids labeling individuals as mentally ill.

4. Which of the following nursing diagnoses reflects the NANDA human response pattern of choosing?

   a. Dysfunctional grieving   Feeling
   b. Ineffective individual coping
   c. Altered role performance   Relating
   d. Chronic low self-esteem   Perceiving

5. The primary purpose of developing a nursing care plan is to:

   a. Help the client set realistic goals.
   b. Identify psychotherapeutic interventions.
   c. Provide health teaching.
   d. Collect client data.

6. During the nursing assessment, the client mentions that he feels ill at ease around people. Which of the following would be the most appropriately stated goal to address this situation?

   a. Client will state a desire to improve his social situation.
   b. Client will not sit alone in his room during group sessions.
   c. Staff will provide opportunities for client to socialize.
   d. Client exhibits impaired social interaction.

7. Which of the following best describes the role of a client advocate for the mentally ill?   CASE MAN.

   a. To coordinate therapeutic support services
   b. To identify mentally ill clients in the community
   c. To educate clients about rights and responsibilities
   d. To provide ongoing psychotherapy

8. Which of the following is one of the most significant advantages of community mental health services?

   a. They promote reintegration of the client into society.
   b. They provide intense supervision of clients.
   c. They are easily accessible to clients.
   d. They rarely let clients "fall through the cracks."

ANSWERS

1. **Correct answer is b.** Neurotransmitters and their role in schizophrenia, affective disorders, and anxiety disorders are a primary focus of current research.

   a. Urban violence is considered a public health problem.
   c. Currently, alcohol dependence is considered a primary disease process.
   d. The parent-child relationship is no longer considered the primary factor in the development of most mental illnesses, particularly psychotic disorders. Family system models do, however, focus on parental roles and family structures as critical factors in individuals predisposed to mental illness.

2. **Correct answer is b.** In the self-help model, individuals with a common disorder come together to offer each other support and advice.

    a. The holistic model is an approach to health care that considers the physical, mental, social, developmental, and spiritual needs of the client.
    c. The cognitive model focuses on the client's thought processes in an attempt to identify negative or dysfunctional thoughts.
    d. Derived from the work of Harry Stack Sullivan, the interpersonal model is based on the idea that personality can be observed and studied only in the context of a relationship with another individual.

3. **Correct answer is c.** The primary advantage of the DSM is that it clearly identifies disorders and symptoms.

    a. One disadvantage of the DSM is that it does not consider social and cultural variables that might have an impact on the presentation of mental disorders.
    b. One disadvantage of the DSM is that the categories are rigid and individual variables are not considered in the diagnostic scheme.
    d. Diagnostic labeling, which is done in DSM, can have a harmful effect on an individual's personal and professional life.

4. **Correct answer is b.** The nursing diagnosis of ineffective individual coping is an example of the NANDA human response pattern of *choosing,* or selecting alternatives.

    a. The nursing diagnosis of dysfunctional grieving is an example of the human response pattern of *feeling,* or having subjective awareness.
    c. The nursing diagnosis of altered role performance is an example of the human response pattern of *relating,* or establishing bonds.

    d. The nursing diagnosis of chronic low self-esteem is an example of the human response pattern of *perceiving,* or receiving information.

5. **Correct answer is a.** During the planning phase of the nursing process, the nurse establishes priorities for care, sets goals with the client, determines outcome criteria, and develops methods for obtaining goals.

    b. Identifying psychotherapeutic interventions is the focus of the implementation phase of the nursing process.
    c. Providing health teaching is part of the implementation phase of the nursing process.
    d. Collecting client data is the focus of the assessment phase of the nursing process.

6. **Correct answer is a.** One of the purposes of client care goals is to translate the client's vague feelings and statements into concrete statements of goals.

    b. Client care goals should be stated in positive terms.
    c. Client care goals should be client focused and should indicate client outcomes.
    d. This statement is the basis of a nursing diagnosis, not a goal or an expected outcome.

7. **Correct answer is c.** Client advocates provide information to clients about their rights and responsibilities as well as working to see that services are made available to clients.

    a. It is the role of the case manager to coordinate outpatient therapeutic services in order to help clients live in the community.
    b. Nurses who undertake case-finding identify people who need treatment for mental health problems. This is not a primary function of client advocates.
    d. Psychotherapists of various backgrounds (e.g., psychiatrists, psychologists, social workers, and clinical nurse specialists) provide psychotherapy. This is not a function for a client advocate.

8. **Correct answer is a.** Clients can participate in a familiar social setting while receiving mental health services.

   b. One disadvantage of community mental health treatment is that the client's activities of daily living cannot be directly supervised.

   c. Community mental health centers normally encompass geographic areas of approximately 100,000 persons. It may be difficult for individuals with a mental illness to travel to and from a central location on a daily or weekly basis.

   d. It is not unusual for clients to drop out of treatment and become lost to the community health services. Clients might relapse or change residence and fail to follow up with their treatment.

2

Models of Psychiatric Care

NURSING HIGHLIGHTS

1. Theories of psychiatric care provide the conceptual framework for treatment; the treatment model will greatly influence the interventions and techniques that are employed.
2. Nursing model complements other treatment models; it does not compete with them or supplant them.
3. Nurse must be familiar with all models of psychiatric care and theories underlying them.
4. Nurse adapts nursing care plan to reflect treatment model that is being used.
5. Many health care providers combine elements of various models of care when developing an individualized treatment plan for the client.

anxiety—vague yet pervasive apprehension that is accompanied by feelings of uncertainty and helplessness

conscious—in Freud's theory, portion of the mind that is aware of surroundings

defenses—coping mechanisms one uses to protect oneself from unpleasant feelings such as anxiety or guilt

deviance—behavior that is significantly different from what is considered normal by a social group

ego—in Freud's theory, an element of personality that distinguishes between the mind and external world

fixation—in psychoanalytic model, failure to develop beyond an early psychosexual stage

free association—therapeutic technique in psychoanalysis in which client verbalizes to therapist all thoughts that come to mind

id—in Freud's theory, source of all drives

neurotic defenses—actions, designed to counteract anxiety, that are inflexible and usually unconscious

neurotransmitter—chemical that allows transmission of an electrical impulse across gap (synaptic cleft) that separates 1 neuron from another; triggers complex biologic reactions in cells

preconscious—in Freud's theory, part of the mind containing experiences, thoughts, and feelings that can be recalled into the conscious but also having the capability to screen out and censor unwanted or unpleasant experiences and thoughts

psychosis—severe mental disorder in which a person experiences dysfunctional behavior with a loss of sense of reality

stressor—any event or situation, positive or negative, that produces a state of physical or emotional tension

superego—in Freud's theory, one's conscience

transference—an unconscious response process in which client projects upon the nurse or other caregivers feelings originally directed to a significant person in the client's past, such as a parent

unconscious—in Freud's theory, part of the mind containing thoughts and memories that are not directly available to the conscious mind but that have significant effect on one's conscious thought and behavior

I. Anxiety model

A. Background

See text pages
_____

1. The anxiety model views behavior as an attempt to relieve or resolve stress.
2. Stress may be caused by physical, psychologic, developmental, emotional, cultural, or social stressors.
3. Stress precipitates an anxiety reaction that may be constructive or destructive.

I. Anxiety model	II. Psychoanalytic model	III. Interpersonal model	IV. Social model	V. Existential model

(handwritten annotations: "Freud. Erikson" above column II; "Jung", "Freud Frieda", "Searles" within/below column II; "H Stack Sullivan" below column III)

B. Principles
1. The anxiety continuum: can be used as a conceptual model for understanding/classifying psychiatric syndromes
   a) Mild anxiety is a positive psychic force that aids in the work of living (e.g., studying for an exam, preparing for a job interview).
   b) Moderate anxiety is exhibited as physical symptoms (e.g., asthma, high blood pressure).
   c) Severe anxiety is exhibited as neurotic defenses.
   d) Severe anxiety/panic is exhibited as personality disorders (e.g., borderline, antisocial, histrionic personalities).
   e) Panic is exhibited as psychosis.
2. Therapy approaches (see Chapter 5, section II)
3. Nurses employ knowledge about the concept of anxiety in planning nursing interventions for clients with many disorders in addition to anxiety disorder (e.g., knowledge that increased anxiety levels negatively affect clear thinking and problem solving).

II. Psychoanalytic model

See text pages
_____

A. Background
1. Sigmund Freud developed complex principles of neurotic human behavior in late 1800s.
   a) Classification of mental operations: conscious, preconscious, unconscious
   b) Structure of mind: ego, id, superego
2. Theory expanded and modified by many other theorists: Erik Erikson (psychosocial stages of development), C. G. Jung (collective unconscious), Anna Freud (psychoanalytic study of children), and Frieda Fromm-Reichmann and Harold Searles (psychoanalytic techniques in treatment of psychosis).

B. Principles
1. Behavior deviations are rooted in childhood developmental stages.
2. Problems arising during developmental stages cause fixations.
3. Later stress causes regression.
   a) To escape difficult problems, one returns psychologically to an earlier stage of development and uses the defenses/coping mechanisms that were effective then.
   b) The client cannot use mature coping techniques because the childhood conflict was never resolved (e.g., a boy who has unresolved feelings toward his mother may later have difficulty establishing relationships with women).
4. Physical symptoms are symbols/metaphors for psychologic distress (e.g., excessive hand-washing is an attempt to symbolically cleanse oneself of actions perceived to be unclean).

5. Therapy (psychoanalysis) is aimed at helping the client recognize and resolve intrapsychic/unconscious conflicts.
    a) Therapy is typically long-term and intensive.
    b) Several methods of treatment are used.
        (1) Free association
        (2) Dream therapy
        (3) Interpretation/guidance by therapist: may cause transference and countertransference
        (4) Hypnosis
6. Role of nurse has been historically limited because treatment is focused on physician or therapist.

III. Interpersonal model

See text pages
_____

A. Background
    1. Theory was established by H. S. Sullivan.
        a) Self-system: Sullivan's term for a person's view of self
        b) Reflected appraisals: means of developing a view of self through experiences learned by interaction with others; may be positive or negative
    2. Interpersonal therapy focuses on social, cultural, and interpersonal factors affecting personality development (as opposed to the intrapsychic factors emphasized in psychoanalysis).

B. Principles
    1. The self is built on and influenced by childhood experiences.
    2. Interpersonal model assumes that humans are motivated by 2 basic needs.
        a) Need for satisfaction (e.g., hunger, lust, loneliness)
        b) Need for security—culturally defined needs, such as conformity; accompanied by fear of rejection
    3. Interpersonal therapy treats the client through the "corrective interpersonal experience."
        a) Healthy relationship with the therapist becomes a model for other successful life experiences.
        b) Therapist shares feelings, thoughts, experiences (as opposed to psychoanalysis, in which the therapist maintains a neutral posture); partnership develops.
    4. Interpersonal therapy contains concepts basic to the interpersonal relationship between psychiatric nurse and client (e.g., that of teacher/learner, empathizer/client, counselor/client, resource provider/consumer).

IV. Social model

See text pages
_____

A. Background
    1. Social model considers social context of client: It defines psychiatric problems in terms of deviance from societal norms.
    2. Social model emphasizes community mental health and broad social programs to prevent or mitigate the root causes of deviance.

Sartre

II. Psychoanalytic model	III. Interpersonal model	IV. Social model _Caplan & Szasz_	V. Existential model _Kierkegaard_ ,	VI. Communication model

3. The 2 main theorists are Gerald Caplan and Thomas Szasz.
    a) Caplan focuses on prevention; he emphasizes social causes of mental illness, such as poverty, family life, poor education.
    b) Szasz defines mental illness as a "myth" (i.e., a true illness is physical, but deviance is a social phenomenon).

B. Principles
    1. The social model applies a social definition of deviance.
        a) "Deviant" behavior is not an objective fact but a judgment imposed by society.
        b) In other cultures, the same behavior may not be considered deviant at all.
    2. Crises are key factors in social model: They can trigger deviant behavior or can be an opportunity for growth, depending on the availability of social supports and the client's development of his/her own coping mechanisms.
    3. Therapy techniques are linked to social environment.
        a) Caplan endorses community mental health programs and emphasizes the need for prevention through improvement of poverty and other social problems; urges action by professionals on a broad continuum, ranging from individual therapy to consultation on social programs.
        b) Szasz advocates client's freedom of choice in selecting a therapist and treatment method; he opposes involuntary hospitalization and other "coercive" measures.
    4. Role of psychiatric nurse is expanded within this model because of shift away from physician-dominated care; nurse's role as teacher and counselor to client and family is utilized.

> See text pages
> _____

V. Existential model

A. Background
    1. Influenced by existential philosophies of Sartre, Kierkegaard, and so on, the existential model emphasizes the here-and-now rather than the client's past experiences.
    2. Existential model assumes that deviant behavior occurs when an individual is alienated from himself/herself or from his/her surroundings.
        a) Alienation from the self causes feelings of sadness, loneliness; interferes with meaningful relationships with others.
        b) Alienation from surroundings causes feelings that life is meaningless, absurd, invalid; leads to lack of commitment.

B. Principles
    1. The existential model emphasizes the "encounter."
        a) An encounter is a shared interaction in which each person acknowledges the "total existence" of the other.

b) It is the basic tool to reestablish the client's connection to the self and surroundings.
2. Existential therapy uses a number of specific approaches to treatment.
   a) Logotherapy: focuses on the "search for meaning" (logos) in the client's life; attempts to help client take control of own life and define its meaning for himself/herself
   b) Gestalt therapy: focuses on the here-and-now, such as the physical sensations that accompany emotions; therapy techniques designed to elicit spontaneous reactions
   c) Rational-emotive therapy: uses confrontation to encourage client to take responsibility for behavior; emphasizes action on part of client and therapist
   d) Encounter group: looks to establish intimate interaction in group settings; emphasizes honest and open sharing of feelings to promote self-awareness
   e) Reality therapy: helps client recognize life goals and what is blocking them; helps develop client's capacity for caring through the client's relationship with therapist; encourages client to focus on behavior rather than feelings

VI. Communication model

See text pages
_____

A. Background
1. The communication model defines behavior as verbal and/or nonverbal communication and deviance as flawed communication.
   a) Clients, spouses, families, and groups are made aware of dysfunctional communication patterns through education and feedback.
   b) Building on this awareness, therapist works with all concerned to create new, more functional patterns of communication.
2. Communication theorists include Eric Berne (transactional analysis), Richard Bandler and John Grinder (neurolinguistic programming), Paul Watzlawick (pragmatics), and Jurgen Ruesch (therapeutic communication).

B. Principles
1. Transactional analysis
   a) Theory postulates that people communicate from 3 ego states, acting as parent, adult, or child in the encounter; defines a unit of communication as a transaction.
   b) There are 3 types of transactions.
      (1) Complementary transactions occur when messages are exchanged appropriately: for example, when a "parent" addresses a "child" and the "child," in turn, responds to the "parent."
      (2) Crossed transactions cause interpersonal communication problems.
      (3) Ulterior transactions occur when communicators have hidden motives; can be destructive.
2. Neurolinguistic programming
   a) Theory focuses on the sensory channels through which people receive information: visual, auditory, and kinesthetic.

IV. Social model	V. Existential model	VI. Communication model	VII. Behavioral model	VIII. Medical-biologic model

b) Theory postulates that each person has a preferred channel through which to send and receive information and an affinity for others who share this preference.

c) Client's preferred channel can be identified from conversational cues (e.g., "See what I mean?" or "Do you hear what I'm saying?") and from actions (e.g., hand movements or eye movements).

d) Therapy is tailored to the individual by using his/her preferred channel (e.g., "Tell me what's on your mind," "You look like you have something to say," or "What are you feeling?").

3. Pragmatic model

a) Theory identifies relationships as either symmetric (equal) or complementary (based on difference).

b) Theory focuses on disrupted communication patterns.

   (1) Efforts not to communicate at all, which is impossible

   (2) Attempts to communicate at levels that are incongruent (e.g., when 1 person is focusing on the factual content of the message and the other on the emotional content)

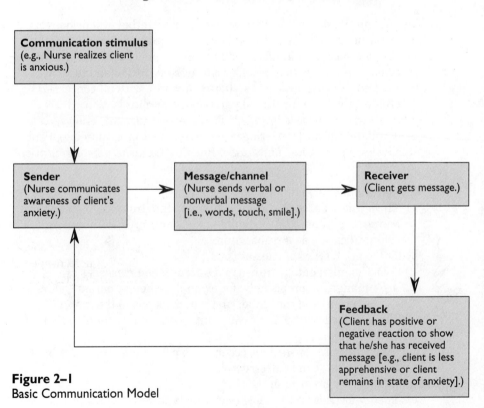

Figure 2–1
Basic Communication Model

(3) Situations in which messages are misunderstood or incorrectly perceived, such as when the listener lacks critical information or holds incorrect assumptions

   c) Change is brought about in therapy through telling the client to change or telling the client not to change.

4. Therapeutic communication

   a) According to this theory, communication is a dynamic process that continues until parties agree to end it or 1 party leaves.

   b) Ability to communicate is based on perception (sensory reception), evaluation (cognitive and affective responses influenced by personal experience), and quality of transmission (feedback).

   c) Based on feedback, communicator refines message.

   d) To be therapeutic, communication must have these qualities: efficiency (with simplicity, clarity, and focus), appropriateness, and flexibility.

5. Facilitative communication strategies

   a) Techniques help initiate and maintain trusting therapeutic relationships.

   b) Skills include:

      (1) Giving information: Nurse gives client needed facts (e.g., about client's therapy or medication schedule); technique should not include giving advice.

      (2) Listening actively.

      (3) Giving broad openings: Nurse lets client know client can choose topic for discussion.

      (4) Restating: Nurse paraphrases what client has said to be sure nurse understands client's comment.

      (5) Clarifying: Nurse asks client to give an explanation or example of a vague comment client has made.

      (6) Reflecting: To show that nurse has heard and understood client's message and to show respect for client's thoughts, nurse repeats in her/his own words client's verbal or nonverbal message.

      (7) Sharing perceptions: Nurse asks client to verify that nurse has understood what client has said or done or is feeling.

      (8) Focusing: Nurse helps client concentrate on 1 issue.

      (9) Identifying theme: Nurse attempts to identify underlying issues—issues that come up repeatedly.

      (10) Using silence: Nurse gives client time to think; nurse can communicate interest nonverbally while waiting for client to speak.

      (11) Summarizing: Nurse lists topics that have been discussed in the current meeting or in a previous meeting.

      (12) Suggesting: Nurse presents alternate ways for client to view a situation.

6. Nursing role: Effective communication is integral to nursing care of psychiatric clients. Communication therapy techniques and strategies may be integrated into assessment and implementation stages of nursing process.

V. Existential model	VI. Communication model	VII. Behavioral model	VIII. Medical-biologic model	IX. Nursing model

See text pages
_____

VII. Behavioral model (see Chapter 3, section VI, for more information on the therapeutic techniques)

A. Background
1. Behavioral therapy was pioneered by B. F. Skinner and others.
2. Theory focuses on external behavior (what happens), not on internal thoughts or feelings (why it happens).
3. Theory emphasizes ability to measure effectiveness of treatment by objective methods.

Skinner

B. Principles
1. Behavior is defined as acts that are quantifiable and measurable.
2. Behavior is learned (e.g., fear of a hot stove resulting from being burned) and reinforced through repetition.
3. Deviant behavior is a result of reinforcement/reward.
4. In therapy, the frequency of dysfunctional behavior is decreased and frequency of desirable behavior is increased.
5. Success of therapy is judged by measurable changes in frequency of identified behavior.
6. Psychiatric nurse uses principles of behavioral model as part of interventions in many areas of practice.

See text pages
_____

VIII. Medical-biologic model

A. Background
1. Theory defines psychiatric problems as a disease process (i.e., central nervous system dysfunction) analogous to physical illness.
2. Theory builds on traditional physician-client relationship.
3. Theory avoids moralistic overtones by not assigning blame to client.
4. Theory studies biochemical bases of emotion, behavior, thought, and mood; also examines genetics and environment.
5. Because model emphasizes biochemical bases of thought and behavioral problems (e.g., malfunctioning of neurotransmitters at synapse receptors in central nervous system), it places great reliance on pharmacotherapy and research into biochemical/neurologic basis for mental illness.

B. Principles
1. Medical-biologic model adopts a therapeutic approach that mirrors medical treatment of physical illness.
   a) Examination and history taking
   b) Formulation of diagnosis
   c) Treatment, planned and coordinated by physician but possibly involving many types of caregivers
   d) Evaluation, both subjective (client's perception) and objective (assessment of function, behavior)
   e) Long-term follow-up care, if indicated

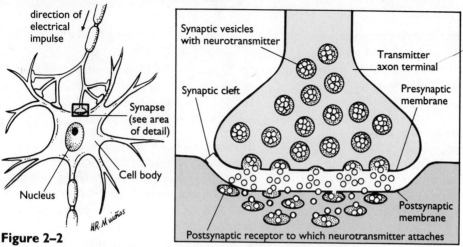

Figure 2–2
Action of Neurotransmitter in Central Nervous System Neurons

2. Essential features of nursing care are knowledge of drug administration, data gathering, and client education to instruct clients and families about psychiatric drugs used in management of disorders.

IX. Nursing model

A. Background

See text pages

1. Nursing diagnosis—as distinct from other care models—is becoming the basic paradigm for assessing and implementing psychiatric nursing care.
2. Many theorists have established nursing models (e.g., H. Peplau, L. Hall, D. Orem).
3. Nursing model is distinct from, yet complements, physician/therapist interventions.
4. Nursing model does not replace other models of care but complements them.
5. Nursing model focuses on client's response to potential or actual health problems.

B. Principles

1. Nursing model employs the nursing process (see Chapter 1, section III).
2. Although definitions are still evolving, basic nursing principles involve elements of holistic care, collaboration between client and nurse to establish relationship, caring role.
   a) Nurse's role is to promote client self-care by compensating for client's inability to care for self and by supporting client.
   b) Nurse works as teacher, counselor, and listener and participates in other interpersonal roles.
   c) Nurse intervenes to help client adapt to demands: physiologic, self-concept, social, and interdependence.

1. Marissa is newly admitted to the psychiatric unit at the local hospital. She recently lost her job and is the sole support of her 3 children. During the interview with the nurse, Marissa paces, is short of breath, and keeps repeating, "I can't stand this, and I have 3 small children." When another client startles her by yelling at the nurse, she paces more rapidly. Marissa is having difficulty focusing on the nurse's questions. The most appropriate assessment of the stage of anxiety is:
   a. Severe anxiety.
   b. Mild anxiety.
   c. Panic.
   d. Moderate anxiety.

2. Marissa continues to become increasingly anxious. The most appropriate communication technique for the nurse to employ at this time is to:
   a. Command Marissa to sit down and gain control of herself.
   b. Whisper in Marissa's ear that everything will be all right.
   c. Stop the interview questions and escort Marissa to the middle of the day room.
   d. Attend to Marissa's behavior, and direct her to a quiet area.

3. Mary, a nurse, has been working in a community mental health center in an urban area for 15 years. Recently, she began calling her state legislators because she believes it is the social conditions that complicate her work. What theorist has best described her beliefs?
   a. Sigmund Freud
   b. Erik Erikson
   c. Gerald Caplan
   d. Sister Callista Roy

4. Jorge is an engineer who often states during his conversations with other clients and with the nurse, "I hear what you're saying." Utilizing principles from neurolinguistic programming, the nurse's most appropriate response would be:
   a. "Listen to what I am saying."
   b. "See what I am illustrating."
   c. "Feel what this arouses."
   d. "Recognize the perception."

5. Monica, who has a problem with excessive dependence, has just talked with her psychiatrist. She looks puzzled and says to the nurse, "Dr. Simpson just told me to be more dependent." The nurse knows that the psychiatrist is utilizing which of the following techniques?
   a. Neurolinguistic programming
   b. Transactional analysis
   c. Therapeutic double bind
   d. Rational-emotive therapy

6. James, a nurse on the chemical dependency unit, has been assigned Chuck, a 19-year-old. Chuck has had numerous hospitalizations for alcohol and chemical abuse. Chuck came in recently after losing his fourth job in 3 months and going on a binge. He binges about every 3 months and has refused disulfiram (Antabuse) as part of his recovery program. James has sought Chuck out, encouraging him to talk today. James's most appropriate opening comment would be:
   a. "I'm assigned to talk with you today. Let's discuss Antabuse."
   b. "I heard you binge every 3 months."
   c. "Don't try to manipulate me today. I didn't like it yesterday."
   d. "I'm assigned to talk with you today. What is it you might like to talk about?"

7. During the conversation with Chuck, James invites Chuck to clarify this vague comment: "Man, nobody knows the gutter like the gutterman." Which of the following statements by the nurse would best invite clarification?
   a. "I know how you feel about the gutter."
   b. "It sounds as if you don't like falling from grace."

c. "Could we go back to your statement about the ward rules?"

d. "Tell me more about being a gutterman in the gutter."

8. As Chuck talks, James recognizes that Chuck is repeatedly giving examples of his lack of control. The nurse's best attempt at identifying a theme is:

a. "Repeat to me what you said yesterday."

b. "I hear you saying life is hard."

c. "Since we have been talking, you have repeatedly described many moments during which you have been out of control."

d. "Controlling your life is very important for survival."

9. Angel is a 22-year-old client who was recently placed on an antidepressant medication. Utilizing a medical-biologic framework, the nurse is responsible for:

a. Intervening with the doctor and expressing a belief in social/learning models.

b. Explaining to the client the specific role of neurotransmitters in most psychiatric disorders.

c. Refusing to administer this medication because its side effects have been debated in the local newspaper.

d. Explaining to the client and her husband general information about the class of drug, the reason the client is taking the drug, and potential side effects.

ANSWERS

1. Correct answer is a. The client is experiencing severe anxiety. She is worrying about her children, a smaller detail than her current loss of control in the immediate setting. She is unable to focus on the nurse, and her anxiety increases when she hears another person yell.

b. If the client were mildly anxious, she would be able to answer the nurse's questions and would not become more agitated when the other client yells.

c. A client at the panic stage of anxiety would be more disordered and unaware of other events in her environment. Communication would be unintelligible, and she would not be able to identify any details of her difficulties, such as having 3 children.

d. A client with moderate anxiety would shut out the yelling patient and be more intently focused on the nurse and her questions. She would not behaviorally display her anxiety by pacing.

2. Correct answer is d. By attending to the client's behavior, the nurse is sending a message to the client that she is concerned and that she is in control. Removing the client to a quiet area will decrease environmental stimuli.

a. A command may increase the client's anxiety; also, the client has minimal voluntary control.

b. A whisper may not be heard by the client. In addition, telling the client at this point that everything will be all right is patronizing and difficult for the client to believe.

c. Stopping the interview is correct, but putting Marissa in the middle of the day room will increase the environmental stimuli, which will increase her anxiety.

3. Correct answer is c. Caplan's theory included the client's social environment and prevention activities. By recognizing the social conditions, Mary is attending to the environment; by advocating with legislators, she is utilizing prevention.

a. Mary would attend more to the intrapsychic functioning of the individual if she were using Freud's theory.

b. Mary would attend more to developmental stages and tasks of the individual if she were using Erikson's theory.

d. Mary would attend more to how clients' adaptive or maladaptive responses were displayed if she were using the theory of Roy.

4. **Correct answer is a.** Jorge's preferred mode is auditory, which is reflected in his statement, "I hear what you're saying." By utilizing the auditory cues "listen" and "saying," the nurse is responding in an auditory fashion.

    b. The cues "see" and "illustrate" denote a visual style of response.
    c. The cues "feel" and "arouses" denote a kinesthetic style of response.
    d. The cues "recognize" and "perception" denote a visual style of response.

5. **Correct answer is c.** Therapeutic double bind utilizes paradoxic communication with the client to increase the client's awareness and anxiety and to stimulate the client to change.

    a. Neurolinguistic programming utilizes congruent predicates and involves matching the therapist's communication style to that of the client.
    b. Transactional analysis utilizes the labeling and analysis of games played in communication.
    d. Rational-emotive therapy helps clients deal with emotional problems by direct confrontation of irrational beliefs.

6. **Correct answer is d.** James gives the client information and then leaves a broad opening to let the client know that he can choose the topic of the communication.

    a. It is important that James let the client know he is assigned to him; however, the client should be allowed to choose the topic for discussion.
    b. James does not state his purpose in talking with the client, and he rapidly chooses the topic of discussion.
    c. The nurse is not showing respect for the client. He states the reason for the interaction and gives feedback at an inappropriate time during the communication.

7. **Correct answer is d.** The nurse is clear and is inviting the client to be more specific about the meaning of the statement.

    a. The nurse is attempting to be empathetic, but the statement may have 1 meaning for the client and another meaning for the nurse.
    b. The nurse is attempting to interpret the client's statement with a statement that is very vague.
    c. The nurse is attempting to focus, not to clarify.

8. **Correct answer is c.** This describes the nurse's observation and summary of a repetitive theme.

    a. The nurse is attempting to point out a pattern, but this statement is too vague and broad.
    b. The nurse is interpreting what the client has said but does not point out repetitive themes.
    d. The nurse acknowledges a theme but is giving advice, not pointing out the theme to the client.

9. **Correct answer is d.** The nurse is responsible for appropriate education about medication in the medical-biologic model of treatment.

    a. A nurse working within a medical-biologic model may discuss an opinion with the physician, but the nurse has a responsibility to carry out the physician's order if it is common practice and sound.
    b. A nurse has a role to educate the client, but much is unknown about the specific roles of neurotransmitters. This discussion is too broad to be relevant to an individual client.
    c. A nurse may refuse to administer an inappropriate dosage of a medication or a medication that is contraindicated due to interaction with other medications, the physical condition of the client, or known allergies. It would not be sound professional judgment to refuse administration based on reports in the lay media.

3

Therapies and Interventions

1. Nurse must be familiar with a variety of therapies and interventions.
2. Therapies and interventions are not mutually exclusive; a client's treatment plan may use a variety or combination of therapies and interventions.
3. Nurse should develop nursing plans that reflect the goals and methods of treatment.
4. Essential to psychiatric nursing practice is the continuing interpersonal therapeutic nurse-client relationship.
5. In therapeutic relationships, nurse works in a goal-directed manner to assist clients in making useful changes in their lives.
6. Psychiatric interventions and therapies may be applicable to a variety of nursing tasks in nonpsychiatric settings, such as client education and relief of anxiety.

GLOSSARY

adaptive behavior—any measurable, observable act, movement, or response that enables an individual to adjust to the environment

catharsis—therapeutic release of anxiety or stress brought about by facing and discussing a problem

developmental tasks—fundamental physical, social, intellectual, and emotional behaviors that must be acquired at each age or stage of life in order to achieve normal and healthy development

empathy—ability of a nurse to objectively experience the feelings, thoughts, and attitudes of a client in order to understand these entities on the client's terms

maladaptive behavior—any act, movement, or response that is detrimental to the actor or to those around the actor; an ineffective coping mechanism

polypharmacy—use of combinations of drugs to treat psychiatric disorders

psychotropic drug—drug that has a mind-altering effect

somatic therapy—therapy that uses physical measures to treat psychiatric conditions

therapeutic alliance—conscious contractual relationship in which therapist aligns himself/herself with the reality-oriented and growth-directed aspects of a client's personality to help the client and the therapist understand the client's problems

token economy—behavior modification technique that uses desired objects as rewards for positive changes in behavior

I. One-to-one relationship between psychiatric nurse and client: on a continuum from informal relationship to formal psychotherapy

See text pages

A. Features of one-to-one therapeutic relationship
1. Mutually defined
2. Goal-directed
3. Collaborative: formation of therapeutic alliance in which nurse therapist and client establish a partnership and a commitment to work together

B. Therapeutic use of self: ability of psychiatric nurse to use clinical techniques, scientific knowledge, experience, and self-awareness of strengths and weaknesses to help client achieve insight and change in behavior
1. Personal attributes of psychiatric nurse that facilitate therapeutic effectiveness
   a) Healthy self-awareness
   b) Awareness of value system
   c) Empathy: involves identification, incorporation, reverberation, detachment
   d) Moral and ethical integrity
   e) Genuineness (honesty, openness)
2. Elements in nurse-client professional relationship built on nurse's therapeutic use of self: respect for client, being available to client, being spontaneous, giving hope, being accepting, being sensitive

C. Phases of one-to-one therapeutic relationship
1. Orientation: establishing contact, confidentiality; developing trust; formulating a contract; identifying client problems
2. Working: maintenance phase in which nurse and client identify and evaluate specific stressors and behaviors; client is encouraged to do self-assessment; client is encouraged to try out adaptive coping behaviors
3. Termination: end of relationship due to many factors (e.g., reaching goals [correcting communication problems or maladaptive behaviors], reaching an impasse)

D. Hindrances to the one-to-one therapeutic relationship
1. Resistance: Client is reluctant to explore and examine self, does not want to implement change.
   a) Behavior that contributes to resistance
      (1) Client feels pressured to move too quickly.
      (2) Client feels a lack of respect by the therapist.
      (3) Client does not want to give up secondary benefits of illness (e.g., time off from work, sympathy).
      (4) Client feels therapist has explored too deeply.
      (5) Therapist is not proper role model for client.
   b) Manifestations of resistance
      (1) Forgetfulness
      (2) Acting out

I. One-to-one relationship	II. Group therapy	III. Milieu therapy	IV. Family therapy	V. Crisis intervention

(3) Repression or avoidance

(4) Expressions of hopelessness

(5) Transference

c) Interventions to overcome resistance

   (1) Therapist points out and discusses acts of resistance with client, giving specific examples.

   (2) Therapist reevaluates therapeutic goals.

   (3) Therapist and client agree to a revised plan of action and contract.

   (4) Therapist uses facilitative communication techniques of clarification and reflection.

2. Transference: Client unconsciously attributes to therapist qualities and behaviors that were originally associated with a significant person in the client's early life, perhaps because the therapist looks or acts like the person in the past.

a) Behavior that contributes to transference: Client is using transference as a defense mechanism related to sustaining resistance.

b) Manifestations of transference

   (1) Client is inappropriately hostile to or adoring of therapist.

   (2) Client is dependent on therapist.

   (3) Client assigns meaning to therapist-client interactions that are more appropriate to client's past relationships.

   (4) Client wants to spend extra time with therapist.

   (5) Client asks for special concessions from therapist.

c) Interventions to overcome transference

   (1) Therapist discusses acts of transference with client.

   (2) Therapist reevaluates therapeutic goals and contract.

   (3) Therapist and client reestablish a plan of action agreeable to both.

   (4) Therapist decreases frequency of sessions.

   (5) Therapist ends therapeutic relationship.

3. Countertransference: Therapist has inappropriate, intense emotional response to client; may be caused by therapist's personal needs and problems with authority and assertiveness

a) Manifestations of countertransference

   (1) Inappropriate, irrational hostility toward or affection for client

   (2) Irrational anxiety in presence of client

   (3) Preoccupation with client before and after sessions

   (4) Avoiding or extending sessions

   (5) Encouraging client's dependence on therapist

   (6) Having fantasies about client

b) Interventions to overcome countertransference
  (1) Therapist must conduct self-examination.
  (2) Therapist must reevaluate relationship to see what behavior in client causes therapist's overreactions (e.g., client's aggressiveness or dependence).
  (3) Therapist must renew implementation of techniques that are therapeutically effective (e.g., respect for client, empathy, detachment).
  (4) Sessions should be supervised by peer or other professional.
4. Ineffective communication techniques (see also section VI,B,5 of Chapter 2 for facilitative communication techniques)
  a) Reassuring
  b) Giving approval
  c) Disapproving
  d) Rejecting
  e) Belittling
  f) Using clichés
  g) Giving advice
  h) Probing
  i) Avoiding anxiety-provoking topics
  j) Interpreting unconscious meanings
  k) Requesting a reason (e.g., asking why something is happening rather than what is happening)
  l) Blaming an outside force for client's situation

II. Group therapy: therapy in which a therapist or cotherapists direct and interact with a group of 5–10 people who have an interdependent relationship with one another and a shared purpose of helping one another

See text pages
_____

A. Purposes of therapeutic groups
  1. Individuals can accomplish tasks in groups that they cannot achieve on their own.
  2. Groups are particularly effective in treatment of emotional disturbances and substance abuse disorders.
  3. Groups provide a supportive atmosphere in which members can grow.

B. Functions of therapeutic groups
  1. Content function: Individuals share their experience and insights with those who are facing similar challenges.
  2. Process function: Feedback from others helps an individual gain insights and understanding into her or his problems and behavior; groups serve as a "testing ground" for new behaviors and approaches.

C. Stages of group therapy
  1. Pregroup stage: Therapist (group leader) determines group's purpose, establishes meeting place and times, determines criteria for membership, and selects group members.

2. Orientation stage: Therapist orients the group to its task and fosters structure and cohesion.
3. Conflict stage: Group confronts issues of power and control within itself; issues of "pecking order" and "group politics" are discussed; the group asserts independence and begins to look within itself rather than toward the therapist for guidance.
4. Cohesive stage: Group members' sense of attachment to the group and fellow members increases as conflicts are resolved; trust and self-disclosure increase; negative opinions and feelings tend to be suppressed as damaging to the group's cohesiveness and morale.
5. Working stage: Members begin constructive work on the group's tasks.
6. Termination stage: Open groups may continue indefinitely, even when individual members terminate; closed groups (having a fixed membership) usually terminate after goals are achieved.
   a) Premature termination: Member or group terminates before tasks are successfully completed.
   b) Unsuccessful termination: Member or group cannot successfully address tasks.
   c) Successful termination: Member or group achieves the defined goals; even when successful, group members will normally experience loss/grieving over the termination.

D. Roles of group leader
   1. To help identify ground rules (e.g., no smoking, attendance requirements)
   2. To observe and analyze group communication patterns
   3. To observe roles taken by members
   4. To observe power structure
   5. To observe behavior standards group follows
   6. To promote cohesion
   7. To facilitate interactive communication between self and individual members and among members
      a) Fostering independence
      b) Helping group focus on goals

E. Theoretic frameworks of therapeutic groups
   1. Focal conflict model: This model uses conflicts within the group as a therapeutic tool; it assumes that groups will develop unconscious conflicts, which will have meaning for all the members; therapist helps group arrive at solutions.
   2. Communication model: Purpose is to give group members an opportunity to develop effective ways of communicating with others.
   3. Interpersonal model: This model uses interpersonal theory; therapists work at both individual and group levels, applying such tools as transactional analysis to help group members gain insights.

4. Psychodrama: Through use of dramatic techniques, group members are encouraged to act out problematic situations from their past in order to increase understanding of group members' behavior and achieve insights and catharsis.

F. Nurse's function in group therapy
1. Nurses function as group leaders in informal settings such as health teaching and support groups.
2. Psychiatric nurses lead formal therapy groups with advanced training that includes education in group dynamics and in group therapy theory, clinical practice, supervision by and consultation with an expert in the field.

III. Milieu therapy: therapy that uses elements of the client's immediate environment—people, resources (physical setting), and events—to promote the client's optimal functioning; usually practiced in long-term-care facilities

See text pages
_____

A. Areas of behavior stressed in milieu therapy
1. Activities of daily living (eating, washing, etc.)
2. Interpersonal skills
3. Ability to manage life outside an institution

B. Principles on which milieu therapy is based
1. Emphasis on the dignity and value of the individual—the power of clients to positively influence their treatment and their environment
2. Belief in the importance of healthful surroundings to mental health
3. Dependence on the involvement of all levels of therapeutic staff

C. Nurse's function in milieu therapy
1. Nurse is an active partner in therapy and rehabilitation, working with clients to provide and maintain therapeutic environment.
2. Nurse fosters communication with clients.
3. Nurse teaches clients social skills.
4. Nurse works with all members of therapeutic staff to communicate clients' needs.

IV. Family therapy: therapy that treats the family (i.e., the client and significant others) as a single system rather than focusing on individuals

See text pages
_____

A. Family process and dynamics
1. Family systems include individual family members, their communications, and their interactions.
2. Family systems attempt to maintain a dynamic balance; changes in any part of the family dynamic affects all the other parts as well (for example, a conflict between the son and father may change the relationship of the daughter and mother).
3. An individual's problems or symptoms often reflect larger problems within the family dynamic.

4. Families, like individuals, face developmental tasks (i.e., they are faced with challenges and must grow and adapt to meet them).
5. Dysfunctional families devote excessive energy to maintaining family balance and achieving developmental tasks.

B. Approaches used in family therapy
1. Integrative: emphasizes individual as well as family
2. Psychoanalytic: based on Freudian theory
3. Systems: views family as system combining emotional and social relationships
4. Structural: describes family as open system with clear boundaries and rules
5. Interactional: also known as communications approach; focuses on communication and behavior between and among family members
6. Social network: broadens analysis to include others (friends, neighbors, coworkers) who have social ties to the family or family members
7. Behavioral: uses behavior modification approach, adapted for use with families

C. Major components of family therapy
1. Assessment
   a) Should include participation of all family members
   b) May include structured family tasks
2. Contract negotiation
   a) Begins by asking each family member what he/she would like changed in the family
   b) Proceeds by negotiating attainable goals and tools/techniques that family and therapist will use to achieve them
3. Intervention
   a) Helps family members look at here-and-now and influence of past history
   b) Uses structured family tasks

D. Nurse's function in family therapy
1. Nurse uses knowledge of family therapy theories to reduce acute emotional stress of families in medical crisis.
   a) Observes interactions between family members
   b) Allows family members to express fears and concerns
   c) Uses empathetic, nonreactive listening and responding
   d) Answers questions clearly and directly
   e) Provides education about specific ways to handle crisis
2. To be a qualified family therapist requires graduate training in theory and supervised clinical family therapy experience.

V. Crisis intervention: short-term (usually 6 weeks) treatment method designed to help people cope with a crisis; oriented to the here-and-now; an integral part of nursing care

See text pages
_____

A. Nature of a crisis: an internal disturbance caused by a precipitating event, which overwhelms a person's ability to cope
   1. A crisis is triggered by a specific event or series of events.
      a) Precipitating event creates a threat, challenge, perceived loss, or risk of loss.
      b) Event overwhelms the person's normal coping mechanisms.
   2. A crisis is acute (i.e., it is time-limited).
   3. A crisis has 4 phases.
      a) First phase: Anxiety triggers usual coping mechanisms.
      b) Second phase: If coping mechanisms fail, anxiety increases.
      c) Third phase: New coping mechanisms are attempted, or the challenge is redefined in a way that permits old coping mechanisms to work.
      d) Fourth phase: If anxiety is not resolved in the third phase, psychologic disorganization may result.
   4. A crisis may be any of several types.
      a) Maturational (also known as transitional or anticipated) crisis: a crisis occurring as part of the normal passage from 1 developmental stage to another (e.g., passage from adolescence to adulthood) or as a result of change in social status (e.g., marriage, retirement); requires role changes
      b) Situational (also known as unanticipated) crisis: a crisis occurring when an external event disrupts a person's or group's equilibrium (e.g., job change, divorce, sudden illness, death of loved one)
      c) Adventitious crisis: accidental, uncommon, and unexpected catastrophic crisis affecting many people or many areas of life (e.g., natural disaster, war, airplane crash)
      d) Cultural/social crisis: a crisis caused by cultural or social factors, such as job loss, crime, marital infidelity

B. Goals of crisis intervention
   1. To help client cope with the immediate crisis
   2. To resolve the crisis
   3. To return client to precrisis level of functioning
   4. To allow client to attain improved problem-solving skills

C. Nurse's function in crisis intervention
   1. Assessment of the event and the client's ability to cope with it, specifically:
      a) Precipitating event, including what needs are being threatened and when symptoms of disequilibrium first appeared
      b) Client's perception of the event, including whether perception is realistic or distorted and what memories are surfacing
      c) Support systems available to client: Are family and friends available to help?
      d) Previous strengths and coping mechanisms available to client (see Chapter 5, section I,E)

III. Milieu therapy	IV. Family therapy	V. Crisis intervention	VI. Behavior modification	VII. Psycho-pharmacology

2. Nursing diagnoses: include disabling ineffective family coping, ineffective individual coping, altered thought processes, anxiety
3. Planning: done in collaboration with client and people who are significant in client's life; includes defining realistic goals and means to attain them
4. Interventions
   a) Approach levels
      (1) Environmental manipulation: changing the situation in order to provide situational support or to remove stress
      (2) General support: helping client feel that therapeutic team is on her/his side by demonstrating warmth, acceptance, empathy, and caring
      (3) Generic approach: applying standard protocols of treatment to high-risk clients and to groups of people who have the same specific, well-defined problem or crisis (e.g., grief over the loss of a loved one or recovery from a natural disaster)
      (4) Individual approach: developing specific interventions tailored to individual client's needs; requires flexibility and openmindedness on part of therapist
   b) Specific intervention techniques
      (1) Abreaction: asking open-ended questions about the crisis situation to give client the chance to express feelings, thus reducing client's tension
      (2) Clarification: helping client gain understanding of his/her feelings and their role in the development of the crisis
      (3) Suggestion: helping client view nurse as an empathetic helper, to reduce anxiety
      (4) Manipulation: using client's emotions and values in the therapeutic process to help him/her resolve crisis
      (5) Reinforcing healthy, adaptive behavior by giving positive responses to such behavior
      (6) Encouraging adaptive defense mechanisms and discouraging maladaptive defenses
      (7) Raising self-esteem and helping client regain sense of self-worth
      (8) Exploring alternative ways to solve crisis, perhaps by establishing a social network

VI. Behavior modification

See text pages
_____

A. Purposes
1. To change behavior by changing the consequences (rewards, punishments) of that behavior
2. To teach people with maladaptive behaviors to function effectively and appropriately

B. Techniques
    1. Behavior modification techniques may increase or decrease the
       frequency of behavior.
       a) Techniques that increase or maintain behaviors
          (1) Positive reinforcement: adding a consequence that will
              increase the probability of a behavior's occurrence (e.g., Every
              day that a child completes her math exercises, she is given
              extra time at recess, resulting in an increase in the number of
              days per week that the child completes her exercises.)
          (2) Negative reinforcement: removing or forgoing an aversive
              (painful or unpleasant) consequence to "reward" the desired
              behavior (e.g., A worker arrives on time at his job to avoid
              being reprimanded or fired.)
       b) Techniques that decrease frequency of behavior
          (1) Positive punishment: presentation of an aversive stimulus to
              reduce probability of a behavior's recurrence (e.g., A child hits
              his sibling; the sibling hits him back.)
              (a) Positive punishment raises ethical concerns, especially in
                  institutional settings.
              (b) It is used rarely in clinical settings.
          (2) Negative punishment: removing a reinforcer to reduce
              probability of a behavior's recurrence
              (a) Response cost: removing a reinforcer that was previously
                  available (e.g., An adolescent's driving privileges are
                  revoked as a consequence of missing curfew.)
              (b) Time-out: removing a reinforcer for a period of time (e.g., A
                  child throws his toys at a sibling, so his mother places him
                  on a chair and does not permit him to play for a period of
                  time.)
          (3) Extinction: removing reinforcement for a given behavior (e.g.,
              Parents ignore a child's temper tantrums, depriving the child
              of the attention that he previously received.)
    2. Reinforcement schedules (i.e., the schedule according to which
       reinforcements are delivered) affect the rapidity and permanence of
       behavior change.
       a) Interval schedules: A certain amount of time must elapse between
          reinforcements, no matter how many of the designated behaviors
          occur in the interim.
          (1) Reinforcement is presented for the first desired behavior after
              the given period of time has elapsed.
          (2) In a clinical setting, an interval schedule is easier to
              implement and maintain than a ratio schedule, since behavior
              does not require constant monitoring.
          (3) A fixed interval schedule uses a fixed time schedule (e.g., a
              client who is slow to ambulate is checked hourly; if he is out of
              bed, he receives reinforcement).
          (4) A variable interval schedule uses a variable time schedule.

      b) Ratio schedules: The frequency of reinforcement is based on the frequency of the behavior.

        (1) Ratio schedules result in higher response rates and greater resistance to extinction than interval schedules.

        (2) A fixed ratio schedule delivers reinforcers in ratio to the behavior (e.g., a reinforcer is delivered after every 5 times the behavior occurs).

        (3) A variable ratio schedule varies around an average, which can change over time (e.g., reinforcement may begin at an average of once for every 3 behaviors, gradually diminishing to an average of once for every 30 behaviors).

C. Nurse's function in behavior modification

  1. Used by nurses in their roles as planner, teacher, and role model

  2. Process

    a) Define and measure client's maladaptive behavior.

    b) Employ behavior modification techniques to change that behavior.

    c) Observe client's reaction to techniques (e.g., whether techniques act as positive or negative reinforcers).

    d) Select a reinforcement schedule, using techniques that elicit desired response from client.

    e) Be consistent with responses to client's behavior.

VII. Psychopharmacology: drug treatment of psychiatric conditions

See text pages
_____

A. Principles

  1. Psychopharmacology (drug treatment of psychiatric conditions) seeks to treat psychiatric disorders by altering the biochemistry of the brain.

  2. Psychopharmacology complements other psychiatric therapies and interventions.

B. Types of psychotropic drugs

  1. Antipsychotic medications: to treat schizophrenia, organic brain syndrome with psychosis, manic phase of bipolar (manic-depressive) disorder, severe depression with psychosis

  2. Antidepressant medications: to treat chronic or recurrent severe depression, with symptoms of loss of interest, inability to respond to normally pleasurable activities, significant agitation, excessive guilt

  3. Antimania medication (mood stabilizer): to treat acute manic episodes, hypomanic episodes, bipolar (manic-depressive) disorder

  4. Anxiolytic agents: to treat anxiety-related and stress-related conditions

  5. Sedative-hypnotic drugs: to treat insomnia

C. Drug interactions
  1. Processes
     a) 1 drug interferes with ability of second drug to be absorbed, metabolized, or excreted, affecting effectiveness of second drug.
     b) Drugs interact to increase or decrease effects of each drug.
  2. Risk factors
     a) Polypharmacy (combinations of psychotropic drugs to treat 1 condition or combinations of drugs treating concurrent psychiatric and physiologic conditions)
     b) High doses of multiple drugs
     c) Elderly clients
     d) Clients who have history of noncompliance
     e) Clients who have not received adequate medication education

D. General nursing responsibilities (see chapters on individual disorders for specific information about drugs, their therapeutic and adverse effects, and specific nursing process steps)
  1. Assessment/history taking to obtain baseline information and to obtain list of symptoms that may be treated by psychotropic drugs
     a) Physical examination
     b) Laboratory tests
     c) Mental status evaluation
     d) Drug history: psychiatric, nonpsychiatric, over-the-counter, other legal and illegal substances
     e) Medical, psychiatric, family histories
     f) Assessment of family support
  2. Providing client and family with education about the purpose, side effects, and complications of the drug in a clear, concise, organized way
     a) Awareness of client's capacity to learn
     b) Evaluation of effectiveness of teaching
  3. Administering drugs as ordered
  4. Consistently monitoring for side effects, effectiveness (reduction of symptoms), and possible drug interactions (if client is taking more than 1 drug)
  5. Consistently monitoring compliance (see Nurse Alert, "Recognizing Noncompliance with Drug Regimen")

VIII. Other somatic therapies and interventions

See text pages
_____

A. Electroconvulsive therapy (ECT)
  1. In ECT electric current is passed through electrodes applied to 1 or both of client's temporal lobes to artificially induce seizure activity; client has been anesthetized and has received muscle relaxants; procedure is performed by physician.
  2. ECT is controversial because of its side effects and varying reports of efficacy.
     a) ECT may be used if client cannot tolerate antidepressant drugs or when client has not responded to medication.
     b) ECT may be used for acutely suicidal clients and for those who have not used medication long enough for it to be effective.

      c) Possible side effects and complications include transient confusion, short-term memory loss, headache, nausea, incontinence, hypotension, sinus tachycardia, cardiac arrest.

   3. Nurse's function in ECT

      a) Review physician's explanation of procedure, clarifying any misconceptions client and family may still have.

      b) Be sure client (or if client is incapacitated, family member who has legal authority) has signed consent form.

      c) Be sure that emergency equipment (e.g., oxygen, suction, CPR) is available and in working order.

      d) Conduct usual presurgical preparation.

      e) Provide client with postprocedure orientation as needed; use gentle restraints on agitated client.

      f) Provide predischarge teaching to client and family, including medication dosages and explanation about possible continued confusion.

B. Restraints and seclusion

   1. Research is scant on the therapeutic impact (positive or negative) of the use of physical restraints or seclusion (confinement) in psychiatric treatment.

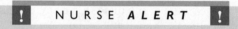

! NURSE *ALERT* !

Recognizing Noncompliance with Drug Regimen

The following factors may increase the likelihood that a client will not comply with medication regimens:

- Failure to establish therapeutic alliance
- Incomplete or inadequate client/family education
- Multiple dosages per day/multiple medications
- Cost/inadequate insurance
- Lack of social supports
- History of noncompliance
- Lack of continuity of care
- Improvement in symptoms—may lead client to feel medication is no longer necessary
- Worsening of symptoms
- Failure to address other stressors/underlying causes of symptoms
- Lack of faith in therapy or team
- Unrealistic expectations
- Unpleasant side effects (e.g., mouth dryness, grogginess, fatigue, dizziness)
- Fear of addiction

2. Physical restraints, which require a physician's order, should be used only when absolutely necessary, after other interventions have failed; preferably they are used for limited time.
3. Indications for restraints include:
    a) Risk of injury to self or others
    b) Ineffectiveness of medication that would control violent behavior or inability to tolerate such medication
    c) Confusion that could result in injury or wandering
    d) Need for rest or for decreased stimuli
    e) Client's request to provide sense of security and control
4. Seclusion or isolation may be necessary for clients who are destructive, violent, or hyperactive.
    a) Seclusion must be used cautiously and never punitively.
    b) Secluded clients require careful monitoring and frequent or continuous observation.
    c) Legal guidelines are scanty and vary from state to state.
    d) Nursing considerations focus on preserving the client's dignity and ensuring fulfillment of basic human needs (e.g., nutrition, cleanliness).

1. At the close of a healthy therapeutic relationship of several weeks' duration, a client brings the nurse a gift of a small craft item, saying, "I want you to have this because I appreciate how much you have helped me." It would be most appropriate for the nurse to say:

   a. "Thank you, but I'm not allowed to accept gifts from clients."

   b. "Thank you. Each time I look at it I will remember the hard work we did together."

   c. "Thank you. You must have known I collect these. It will look nice in my office."

   d. "Your need to give me a gift indicates that we need to spend more time exploring your problems."

2. Which statement by Nurse Jensen about a newly admitted male client might indicate that she is developing countertransference and should reevaluate the relationship?

   a. "This new client looks challenging."

   b. "I'm always a little intimidated by clients like this."

   c. "This client got really angry with me for no reason that I could see."

   d. "All men are alike, and this one really makes me mad for some reason."

3. Nurse Jensen's best response to the development of countertransference would be to:

   a. Continue to build a healthy relationship with the client.

   b. Ask for assignment to another client.

   c. Do more library research on the client's diagnosis.

   d. Discuss her feelings with her supervisor.

4. Ms. Davis has been assigned to a psychotherapy group and asks the nurse why she should participate in the group. The nurse should reply:

   a. "Many goals can be met in a group setting more easily than in an individual setting."

   b. "Group treatment is less expensive than individual therapy."

   c. "You should ask your therapist to reevaluate this decision."

   d. "I think if you try it a few times you will find you like it more than you think you will."

5. Which of the following pieces of information is most important for the nurse to obtain when assessing a client in crisis?

   a. The client's usual coping mechanisms

   b. Available family support or other supports

   c. The client's perception of the problem

   d. The potential for suicide in the client

6. A nurse has been assisting a client throughout a crisis. Which statement by the client indicates the greatest progress toward resolution of the crisis?

   a. "I'm glad I have you to tell me what I should do."

   b. "I've learned several new ways to deal with my problems."

   c. "I'll need to keep seeing you for several years to be really over this."

   d. "I'll never be able to function as well as I did before."

7. Ms. Chin tells the nurse that her 6-year-old son Jon makes her late for work every morning because he procrastinates instead of getting dressed. Which approach should Ms. Chin try first to modify Jon's behavior?

   a. Explain to Jon the importance of being on time for work and school.

   b. Reward Jon with a toy at the end of the week if he is ready on time each day.

   c. Make a chart, and give Jon a sticker each morning that he is ready on time.

   d. Ground Jon to his room each day that he fails to be ready at the set time.

8. Mr. Jingoli was admitted to the psychiatric unit because he was noncompliant with his medication program. The nurse's initial action to deal with this problem should be to:

a. Ask Mr. Jingoli if there is a reason that he failed to take his medication.

b. Explain the importance of regular doses of medication.

c. Obtain orders to administer his medication in liquid form.

d. Find out which family members are available to supervise Mr. Jingoli's medication.

9. Ms. Klidza has received instruction about her psychiatric medications. Which statement by Ms. Klidza indicates a need for more teaching?

a. "I should not stop taking my medication even if my symptoms lessen."

b. "I plan to stop off for beer and pizza on my way home from work."

c. "I don't plan to drive for the next couple of weeks."

d. "This medicine may not cure my disease, but it will make the symptoms more bearable."

10. Which of the following guidelines should be changed to reflect more accurately the philosophy of milieu therapy?

a. All levels of therapeutic staff are involved in the care of the clients.

b. All decisions are made by the attending physician and carried out by the nurse.

c. Clocks, calendars, and newspapers are present on the unit.

d. Nurses maintain open communication with clients and other staff.

ANSWERS

1. **Correct answer is b.** It is appropriate for the nurse to accept a token gift from a client if the client's motive is clear and therapeutic.

a. It is not appropriate for the nurse to accept an expensive gift, but to reject a small gift may be perceived by the client as rejection.

c. The nurse should emphasize the meaning of the gift to the client and the client's feelings, rather than her own.

d. In this situation, the client's offer of a gift is healthy and appropriate.

2. **Correct answer is d.** Countertransference is indicated by strong, irrational feelings that are transferred from previous experience.

a. Perceiving a difficult client as a challenge can be a healthy response by the nurse.

b. Honest expression of feelings by the nurse paves the way for acknowledgment and resolution of difficult feelings.

c. Irrational anger on the part of the client may indicate transference: The client reacts to the nurse out of unresolved conflicts rather than out of the present experiences.

3. **Correct answer is d.** When a nurse has angry or other negative feelings about a client, he/she should initiate a conference with the supervisor to discuss those feelings. Usually, the source of the nurse's feelings can be identified, and the nurse can resolve the countertransference issue and work successfully with the client.

a. Nurse Jensen cannot expect to build a healthy relationship with the client until she resolves the negative feelings.

b. Nurse Jensen should attempt to resolve her feelings through discussion with her supervisor before seeking reassignment.

c. Because the problem is with Nurse Jensen's feelings rather than with her knowledge, library research about the client's diagnosis will probably not be helpful.

4. **Correct answer is a.** Group therapy offers the opportunity to improve social skills, try out new ways of coping, and obtain feedback and support from others who may have similar experiences and feelings. These aspects of group therapy are not easily obtained in individual therapy.

b. Group therapy may or may not be less expensive than individual therapy. The value of group therapy is in the support it may provide the client.

c. This is not an appropriate suggestion for the nurse to make; in addition, statements that begin with "You should . . ." are rarely therapeutic.

d. This response does not address the client's question regarding the rationale for the use of group therapy.

5. **Correct answer is d.** It is most important to ensure the client's physical safety, including assessment for suicide potential.

   a, b, and **c.** These are important, but they do not affect the client's physical safety and thus are lower priority.

6. **Correct answer is b.** Successful intervention leaves the client with new methods of coping with problems.

   a. Early in crisis intervention, it may be necessary for the nurse to give specific directions to the client, but control and responsibility should be returned to the client as soon as possible.
   c. Crises and crisis intervention are time-limited. Crisis intervention usually lasts about 6 weeks.
   d. Successful crisis intervention returns the client to his/her previous level of functioning; if the client has learned new ways of coping, he/she may function even better than before the crisis.

7. **Correct answer is c.** Positive reinforcement that includes immediate, concrete rewards helps reinforce desired behaviors.

   a. Behaviors such as procrastination usually do not reflect a lack of knowledge but rather a need for attention.
   b. A week is too long a time span for a child this age; his positive reinforcement should be immediate and visible. In addition, rewards do not have to be large or expensive as long as the individual perceives them as rewarding.
   d. Negative reinforcement should be avoided. Grounding is inappropriate; the consequence must be related to the incident to be effective.

8. **Correct answer is a.** Clients fail to take medication properly for a variety of reasons. Some common problems include lack

of resources to obtain a supply of medication, lack of understanding about how the medication is to be taken, lack of knowledge about the illness and its treatment, and denial of the need for medication. The nurse must assess the reason before interventions can be planned.

   b. This intervention would be helpful if the client demonstrates a knowledge deficit, but more information is needed before planning interventions.
   c. There are no data yet to suggest that this intervention is appropriate, and it will not insure compliance once the client is discharged.
   d. There are no data yet to suggest that this intervention will be effective for this client. If the problem is denial of the illness and of the need for medication, this intervention may just create family conflict.

9. **Correct answer is b.** Clients taking any kind of psychiatric medications should avoid the use of alcohol, which potentiates central nervous system (CNS) depression.

   a. This is a correct statement. Clients should not stop taking any medication unless they consult their doctor. Some psychiatric drugs, such as benzodiazepines and tricyclic antidepressants, produce withdrawal symptoms when stopped suddenly.
   c. Most psychiatric medications cause drowsiness in the initial period of therapy; clients should not drive or attempt other tasks requiring alertness until they have determined how the medicine affects them.
   d. Medications that cure (remove the disease process) are not yet available for most psychiatric illness. The medications that are available alleviate symptoms and allow many clients to enjoy a better quality of life.

10. **Correct answer is b.** In milieu therapy, decisions are made by the unit group as a whole rather than by any 1 team member. Team decisions are involved.

    a, c, and **d.** These are accurate characteristics of the philosophy of milieu therapy.

4

Assessment Tools

NURSING HIGHLIGHTS

1. Accurate assessment is the foundation for planning, implementing, and evaluating effective psychiatric nursing care.
2. Psychiatric nursing assessment uses a holistic approach, collecting information about all aspects of a client and his/her condition.
3. Data collected by the nurse in the psychiatric nursing assessment amplify and reinforce assessments conducted by other members of the mental health team.
4. Information gathered during the psychiatric nursing assessment and throughout other phases of the nursing process must be documented in writing.
5. Nurse must be aware of his/her personal response to a client during an interview.

I. Psychiatric nursing history	II. Mental status examination	III. Biologic assessment	IV. Psychologic testing	V. Psychosocial assessment

6. Essential elements of the psychiatric nursing assessment are the psychiatric history and the mental status examination; information from biologic and psychosocial assessment and from psychologic testing are also employed by psychiatric nurses in making nursing diagnoses and planning and implementing nursing care.
7. Axes IV and V of DSM-III-R and DSM-IV are particularly valuable in carrying out steps in the nursing process for the psychiatric client.
8. Nurse must safeguard the privacy and legal rights of the client while collecting and using data.

GLOSSARY

affect—any expression of feeling or emotion

compulsion—recurring uncontrollable impulse to perform a certain irrational action

confabulation—invented memories client may use to replace those he/she cannot remember

delusion—fixed false belief or system of beliefs

demographic data—statistical information acquired through study of human populations, including geographic distributions and sex and age distributions

hallucination—sensory experience in the absence of external stimuli

looseness of associations—illogical stream of thought

nihilistic delusion—false belief that the self, part of the self, or another no longer exists

obsession—thought, image, or impulse (usually irrational) that persists in the consciousness against the individual's will

sensorium—an individual's sensory and perceptual mechanism

SOAP note—progress note made on a problem-oriented medical record; includes subjective data, objective data, assessment, plan

somatic delusion—false belief that part or all of the body is impaired

ENHANCED OUTLINE

I. Psychiatric nursing history

See text pages
_____

A. Purposes
1. To assess client's perceptions and memories
2. To provide context for the client's current problem
3. To build rapport with client
4. To help formulate nursing diagnosis and care plan

B. Data collection method and sources
1. Method: interview
2. Sources
   a) Primary source: client
   b) Secondary sources: family, friends, neighbors, police, psychiatric professionals

C. Data collection categories
1. Presenting problem: Quote verbatim from client, if possible; otherwise, construct from other information.
   a) Date of onset
   b) Duration of problem
   c) Present symptoms (physical and behavioral)
   d) Perceived cause of problem, according to client
2. Medical history
   a) Previous illnesses and injuries
   b) Previous hospitalization or treatment
   c) Medication history
   d) Current illnesses, injuries, prescription and over-the-counter medications, and treatment
3. Family history
   a) Psychiatric histories of family members
   b) Family constellation
   c) Family genogram
   d) Home environment
   e) Family roles
   f) Sociocultural family context
   g) Socioeconomic context
   h) Family health status (physical, developmental, psychiatric)
4. Personal history
   a) Demographic and vital data
   b) Birth and development
   c) School history, including achievements, problems
   d) Occupational history
   e) Sexual history
   f) Marital history
   g) Drug use and abuse history, including alcohol, tobacco, illegal and prescription drugs
   h) Religious practices
   i) Interpersonal relationships
   j) Social activities, interests, hobbies

II. Mental status examination

A. Purposes
1. To identify client's current mental status; is not a history
2. To provide objective data to help formulate diagnosis, prognosis, treatment plan

B. Data collection method and sources: observation of client

See text pages
_____

C. Data collection categories
1. General assessments
   a) Behavior
      (1) Echopraxia: imitation of another's movements
      (2) Echolalia: repetition of words and phrases spoken by another
      (3) Akathisia: inability to sit down or lie still
      (4) Dyskinesia: involuntary muscle activity, such as tics or spasms
      (5) Speech patterns (e.g., speed, loudness, flow, intelligibility)
   b) Appearance (physical characteristics, demeanor, hygiene, dress, general health)
   c) Reactions/responses to interview (e.g., cooperative, hostile, passive, agitated)
2. Assessment of client's emotional state
   a) Uses subjective data from the client (e.g., "Client reports, 'I feel scared.'")
   b) Records accompanying objective data (e.g., tears, flushing, foot-tapping)
   c) Notes specific emotional cues
      (1) Intense emotional reaction to specific topics
      (2) Shallowness or flattening of affect in response to specific topics
      (3) Inappropriate emotional responses (e.g., laughing while discussing grief-related topics)
      (4) Simulation (play-acting): intentionally feigned emotions; may be difficult to detect
3. Assessment of thought processes through observations of client's verbal and nonverbal responses, including:
   a) Mutism: Client is aware of questions but does not respond.
   b) Circumstantiality: Client provides overly detailed or convoluted responses.
   c) Perseveration: Client involuntarily repeats words or movements.
   d) Flight of ideas: Client exhibits stream of consciousness speech patterns, including rhyming, punning, and linking phrases through chance associations of words or phrases.
   e) Blocking: Client exhibits sudden, unexplained silences, often due to intrusion of hallucinations or delusions.
   f) Neologisms: Client makes up words whose meanings are known only to the client.
   g) Word salad: Client uses combinations of words and phrases that have no meaning.
4. Assessment of client's thought content
   a) Reality orientation
      (1) Purpose is to establish client's orientation in time, place, person, self, and situation.
      (2) Assessment is performed by asking client to name such things as the month, year, and his/her own name.

b) Preoccupations, including:
    (1) Delusion of persecution ("People have it in for me.")
    (2) Alien control ("Other people can control my thoughts.")
    (3) Nihilistic delusion ("Nothing is real"; "I have no head.")
    (4) Self-deprecation ("I am ugly.")
    (5) Delusion of grandeur ("I am rich, powerful, and influential.")
    (6) Somatic delusion ("I know I have cancer, even though my doctor won't tell me.")
    (7) Hallucinations ("I hear voices"; "I feel bugs crawling on my skin.")
    (8) Obsession ("An earthquake is going to destroy my house.")
    (9) Compulsion (e.g., washing one's hands 50 times a day even when they are not dirty)
    (10) Fantasies and daydreams ("Someday my father will return.")
c) Memory
    (1) Recall of remote past
    (2) Recall of recent past
    (3) Recall and retention of immediate impressions
    (4) General grasp and recall (e.g., ability to remember details and themes after reading a story)
d) General intellectual level
    (1) Grasp of facts: ability to answer general questions (e.g., "Name 5 state capitals.")
    (2) Calculation ability: ability to solve simple arithmetic problems
    (3) Reasoning and judgment: ability to answer such questions as, "If you had $10,000, what would you do?"
e) Abstract thinking, often assessed by asking client to explain the meaning of 1 or more proverbs (e.g., "A rolling stone gathers no moss.")
f) Ability to concentrate: ability to subtract 7 from 100 and to continue as long as able (serial 7s test)
g) Insight: ability of the client to understand his/her psychiatric problems and need for treatment
5. Summary
   a) Findings
   b) Tentative diagnosis

D. Selected standardized mental status assessment tests
1. Mental Status Questionnaire: 10 questions to measure orientation, memory, and general knowledge
2. Short Portable Mental Status Questionnaire: 10 questions to measure orientation, memory, practical skills, and ability to do subtraction
3. Mini-Mental State Examination: measure of orientation, registration, attention and calculation, recall, and language

III. Biologic assessment

See text pages
_____

A. Purposes
1. To identify possible physical causes for a client's psychiatric problem
2. To identify physical disease that may be a contributing or exacerbating factor in the client's psychiatric problem

3. To identify physical problems resulting from the client's psychiatric problem

B. Data collection methods
   1. Biologic history taking
      a) History of known physical diseases and dysfunctions
      b) History of specific physical complaints
      c) Occupational history to uncover possible workplace exposures
      d) Medication (prescription and over-the-counter) client is currently taking
      e) Family history of physical and psychiatric disorders

---

Mini-Mental State Examination

	Maximum score	Score
Orientation		
What is the (year) (season) (date) (day) (month)?	5	(_____)
Where are we (state) (county) (town) (hospital) (floor)?	5	(_____)
Registration		
Name 3 objects: I second to say each. Then ask the patient all 3 after you have said them. Give I point for each correct answer. Then repeat them until he learns all 3. Count trials and record.	3	(_____)
_____ Trials		
Attention and calculation		
Serial 7s. I point for each correct. Stop after 5 answers. Alternatively spell "world" backwards.	5	(_____)
Recall		
Ask for the 3 objects repeated above. Give I point for each correct.	3	(_____)
Language		
Name a pencil, and a watch. (2 points)	9	(_____)
Repeat the following "No ifs, ands, or buts." (I point)		
Follow a 3-stage comment:		
"Take a paper in your right hand, fold it in half, and put it on the floor." (3 points)		
Read and obey the following:		
Close your eyes. (I point)		
Write a sentence. (I point)		
Copy design. (I point)		
	TOTAL SCORE	_____

Assess level of consciousness along a continuum

Alert	Drowsy	Stupor	Coma

SOURCE: Reprinted from Folstein, M. F., S. E. Folstein, and P. R. McHugh. 1975. *Journal of Psychiatric Research* 12:189. Copyright © 1975 by Pergamon Press Ltd. Reprinted by permission of Pergamon Press Ltd.

Figure 4–1
Mini-Mental State Examination

2. Observation
   a) Uneven gait may suggest drug use or brain disease.
   b) Asymmetry (dragging a leg or arm) may suggest brain tumor, stroke.
   c) Poor personal hygiene may suggest emotional disorders or organic brain disease.
   d) Tics and rapid movements may suggest anxiety, chorea, or hyperthyroidism.
   e) Tremors may suggest Parkinson's disease.
   f) Confusion and hallucination may suggest hypoglycemia.
   g) Weight loss may suggest schizophrenia, depression, or physical disorders such as cancer or gastrointestinal diseases.
3. Diagnostic procedures
   a) Neurologic assessment: required for clients who may have organic brain disorder
      (1) Preliminary evaluation
         (a) Pupil reaction time and size
         (b) Level of consciousness
         (c) Ability to respond to various levels of verbal and physical stimuli
         (d) Motor responses
      (2) Electroencephalogram (EEG)
      (3) Computed tomography (CT) scan
      (4) Lumbar puncture
   b) Blood tests to determine presence and level of drugs

IV. Psychologic testing

See text pages
_____

A. Intelligence tests
   1. Stanford-Binet Test
   2. Wechsler Adult Intelligence Scale
   3. Wechsler Intelligence Scale for Children
   4. Gesell Developmental Schedules
   5. Vineland Social Maturity Scale

B. Personality tests
   1. Rorschach Test: uses abstract inkblots to elicit client's thoughts and feelings
   2. Thematic Apperception Test (TAT): uses pictures of people in ambiguous situations to elicit stories reflecting client's emotional state
   3. Minnesota Multiphasic Personality Inventory (MMPI): uses 550 questions related to 9 conditions (e.g., depression, schizophrenic features, hysteria); has standard scoring system
   4. Draw-a-Person Test: asks client to draw human figures; interpretation is based on placement, size of figures, features, etc.
   5. Sentence Completion Test: asks client to complete incomplete sentences; responses are evaluated for insights into client's hopes, fears, etc.
   6. Bender-Gestalt Test: asks client to draw geometric designs that were previously shown to him/her; used to evaluate memory, mental function, and, among children, maturity and motor skills

See text pages
_____

V. Psychosocial assessment

A. Purpose: To provide a continual and holistic assessment of the client and her/his social environment

B. Data collection methods and sources
   1. Methods: interview and observation
   2. Sources: client, family, community

C. Data collection categories
   1. Physical and intellectual assessment
   2. Socioeconomic factors (e.g., employment, cultural and religious factors)
   3. Personal values and goals
   4. Adaptive functioning (e.g., appearance, relationships, communication skills)
   5. Developmental factors (e.g., developmental history, ability to deal with past conflicts)

See text pages
_____

VI. Medical diagnosis (DSM-III-R) (fourth revised edition, DSM-IV, is proposed for publication in 1994)

A. Characteristics
   1. DSM-III-R and DSM-IV are objective.
      a) They use specific numeric codes and names for all recognized mental disorders.
      b) They establish specific diagnostic criteria that must be met for each disorder.
   2. DSM-III-R and DSM-IV are multiaxial.
      a) They increase reliability of evaluations conducted by different clinicians by requiring the clinicians to consider all aspects of a client's condition regardless of their own predilections and theoretic orientation.
      b) They foster a holistic approach to care by incorporating social as well as clinical factors.
      c) They evaluate clients along 5 axes (i.e., in 5 distinct categories, each dealing with a specific class of information).
      d) First 3 axes include elements of the diagnosis to be formulated for every client under psychiatric care; last 2 axes are discretionary.

B. Elements
   1. Axis I: clinical syndromes and other conditions that may be a focus of clinical attention (DSM-IV)
      a) "Other conditions" refers to conditions not attributable to a mental disorder but that are a focus of attention or treatment, such as marital problems or work-related problems.
      b) Axis I includes all psychiatric conditions and associated disorders that are not covered in Axis II.

c) Axis I generally incorporates severe psychiatric conditions, such as alcohol dependence, schizophrenia.

d) Axis I includes code for unspecified mental disorder (i.e., disorder that cannot be classified yet, due to lack of information or other reasons).

e) In DSM-III-R, Axis I is called clinical syndromes and V codes.

2. Axis II: personality disorders (DSM-IV)

a) Axis II reports personality disorders and also includes maladaptive personality features that do not meet the criteria for a personality disorder.

b) Axis II also focuses on defense mechanisms.

c) In DSM-III-R, Axis II is called personality and developmental disorders.

3. Axis III: general medical conditions (DSM-IV)

a) Axis III records and classifies physical disorders and conditions that are relevant to treatment or diagnosis.

b) Axis III may include, for example, conditions such as epilepsy (relevant to potential drug treatments) and history of asthma (relevant to etiology of anxiety).

c) In DSM-III-R, Axis III is called physical disorders and conditions.

4. Axis IV: psychosocial and environmental problems (DSM-IV)

a) Problem categories have been developed to reflect societal changes.

b) Types of problems include those involving primary support group (e.g., death in the family), housing (e.g., homelessness), education (e.g., problem with a teacher), and the law (e.g., being a crime victim).

c) In DSM-III-R, Axis IV is called severity of psychosocial stressors.

5. Axis V: global assessment of functioning (DSM-III-R and DSM-IV)

a) Axis V rates overall level of functioning of client.

b) Axis V rates 3 areas of functioning.

(1) Psychologic

(2) Social

(3) Occupational

c) Global Assessment of Functioning (GAF) Scale is usually for time during which client evaluation is occurring but may also be used to assess functioning for a few months during the previous year.

VII. Documentation

See text pages
_____

A. When information should be recorded

1. At initial contact (i.e., during psychiatric nursing history and mental status examination)

2. At specific intervals throughout treatment (e.g., after each shift or every 24 hours, depending on institutional policy); may have to be done more frequently (e.g., when changes in behavior require immediate intervention)

3. During or after nurse-client interactions (e.g., following therapy sessions, family counseling, client education); done to record overview of interactions

4. At the termination of contact (i.e., at the conclusion of treatment or at discharge or transfer of client)

B. Methods of recording information (see Nurse Alert, "Client Records and the Law")
1. Source-oriented recording
   a) Follows traditional chronologic format
   b) Records physician's and nurse's notes separately
   c) Does not convey integrated view of client care
2. Problem-oriented recording
   a) Developed as an alternative to source-oriented recording
   b) Organizes data to promote better assessment and care: Each member of care team records notes chronologically.
   c) Contains 4 basic elements
      (1) Data base: all information obtained during initial contact
      (2) Problem list: summary of client's problems and assets; continually updated to reflect client's current status
      (3) Initial plans: treatment plans, linked to the problems in the problem list
      (4) Progress notes
         (a) Refer to items on the problem list, detailing client's progress in treatment

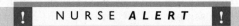

! NURSE *ALERT* !

Client Records and the Law

The clinical records you keep—for example, progress notes and assessment forms—are part of your client's medical records. Observe the following rules regarding records:
- Your client has the legal right to review his/her medical record at any time. If your client wishes to see the chart, go over it with him/her or refer the client to the attending physician. If the client wishes to obtain a copy of the chart, refer him/her to the medical records department.
- The client's record is confidential. Don't divulge its contents to anyone other than mental health team members without the written permission of client. Refer requests for the record to your institution's medical records office or legal office.
- Follow your institution's policies for timely record keeping.
- Don't make changes to the record after the fact, except in accordance with institutional policy; otherwise, you may leave yourself and your institution open to legal liability in the event of a malpractice suit. If you find an error in the chart, no matter how insignificant, don't erase it. Cross it out, and initial and date the correction. Note the change in your progress notes as well.
- Don't express personal opinions and value judgments in the record. Keep it objective and professional.

Global Assessment of Functioning (GAF) Scale[1]

Consider psychological, social, and occupational functioning on a hypothetical continuum of mental health–illness. Do not include impairment in functioning due to physical (or environmental) limitations.

Code (Note: Use intermediate codes when appropriate, e.g., 45, 68, 72.)

100 – 91	Superior functioning in a wide range of activities, life's problems never seem to get out of hand, is sought out by others because of his many positive qualities. No symptoms.
90 – 81	Absent or minimal symptoms (e.g., mild anxiety before an exam), good functioning in all areas, interested and involved in a wide range of activities, socially effective, generally satisfied with life, no more than everyday problems or concerns (e.g., an occasional argument with family members).
80 – 71	If symptoms are present, they are transient and expectable reactions to psychosocial stressors (e.g., difficulty concentrating after family argument); no more than slight impairment in social, occupational, or school functioning (e.g., temporarily falling behind in school work).
70 – 61	Some mild symptoms (e.g., depressed mood and mild insomnia) OR some difficulty in social, occupational, or school functioning (e.g., occasional truancy, or theft within the household), but generally functioning pretty well, has some meaningful interpersonal relationships.
60 – 51	Moderate symptoms (e.g., flat affect and circumstantial speech, occasional panic attacks) OR moderate difficulty in social, occupational, or school functioning (e.g., no friends, unable to keep a job).
50 – 41	Serious symptoms (e.g., suicidal ideation, severe obsessional rituals, frequent shoplifting) OR any serious impairment in social, occupational, or school functioning (e.g., no friends, unable to keep a job).
40 – 31	Some impairment in reality testing or communication (e.g., speech is at times illogical, obscure, or irrelevant) OR major impairment in several areas, such as work or school, family relations, judgment, thinking, or mood (e.g., depressed man avoids friends, neglects family, and is unable to work; child frequently beats up younger children, is defiant at home, and is failing at school).
30 – 21	Behavior is considerably influenced by delusions or hallucinations OR serious impairment in communication or judgment (e.g., sometimes incoherent, acts grossly inappropriately, suicidal preoccupation) OR inability to function in almost all areas (e.g., stays in bed all day; no job, home, or friends).
20 – 11	Some danger of hurting self or others (e.g., suicide attempts without clear expectation of death, frequently violent, manic excitement) OR occasionally fails to maintain minimal personal hygiene (e.g., smears feces) OR gross impairment in communication (e.g., largely incoherent or mute).
10 – 1	Persistent danger of severely hurting self or others (e.g., recurrent violence) OR persistent inability to maintain minimal personal hygiene OR serious suicidal act with clear expectation of death.
0	Inadequate information.

[1]The GAF Scale is a revision of the GAS (Endicott J, Spitzer RL, Fleiss, et al: The Global Assessment Scale: A procedure for measuring overall severity of psychiatric disturbance. *Archives of General Psychiatry* 33:766–771, 1976) and the CGAS (Shaffer D, Gould MS, Brasic J, et al: Children's Global Assessment Scale (CGAS). *Archives of General Psychiatry* 40:1228–1231, 1983). These are revisions of the Global Scale of the Health-Sickness Rating Scale (Luborsky L: Clinicians' judgments of mental health. *Archives of General Psychiatry* 7:407–417, 1962).

SOURCE: Reprinted with permission from the *DSM-IV Draft Criteria (3/1/93)*. Copyright © 1993 American Psychiatric Association.

Figure 4–2
GAF Scale, Axis V

   (b) Use "SOAP" format
      i) S: subjective data, such as client's or family's verbal comments (e.g., "I feel nervous today.")
      ii) O: objective data, such as nurse's observation of behavior (e.g., "Client tapped foot repeatedly during interview.") and physical data (e.g., height, weight, test results)

        iii) A: assessment, the interpretation of the subjective and objective data (e.g., "Client's anxiety appears to be increasing since admission, possibly as a result of upcoming operation.")

        iv) P: plan, the intended course of action for the plan (e.g., "The nursing staff will give client opportunities to express his feelings.")

3. Interaction process analysis (IPA): verbatim recording of verbal and nonverbal interactions between client and nurse

  a) Purposes

    (1) To provide others—consultants, students, other practitioners—with objective data

    (2) To develop the nurse's observation, data collection, and communication skills and planning

    (3) To facilitate review of treatment

    (4) To help nurses assess their own skills and behavior

  b) Components

    (1) Nurse's verbal and nonverbal communication

    (2) Nurse's internal thoughts and feelings

    (3) Intent of the nurse's communication

    (4) Client's verbal and nonverbal communication

    (5) Nurse's interpretation of the client's emotions and intent

    (6) Analysis and interpretation of the communication

    (7) Nursing interventions applied and the rationale for using them

    (8) Evaluation of the interventions' effectiveness

  c) Methods

    (1) On-the-spot recording

      (a) Notes taken during the interaction

      (b) Assures accuracy and completeness

      (c) Has potential for interfering with the interaction

    (2) After-the-fact recording

      (a) Should occur as soon as possible after the interaction

      (b) Preserves spontaneity of the interaction

      (c) Usually results in less complete and accurate data

    (3) Tape recording

      (a) Uses audiotape (most common) or videotape

      (b) Provides complete and accurate record

      (c) May be inhibiting to nurse and/or client

      (d) May be costly or time-consuming to transcribe data

      (e) May result in poor-quality recording

      (f) Requires consent of client

1. When a psychiatric client is preoccupied, avoids eye contact, and laughs inappropriately, the nurse should assess for:

   a. Phobias.
   b. Auditory hallucination.
   c. Flight of ideas.
   d. Loose associations.

2. The nurse uses the proverb "A rolling stone gathers no moss" to evaluate abstract thinking. Which of the following best demonstrates abstract thinking on the part of a psychiatric client?

   a. "You can't stop a stone from rolling away."
   b. "Moss won't grow on a stone."
   c. "If you move around, you never make friends."
   d. "You can never put moss on a rolling stone."

3. A typical plan section of a SOAP note might be expressed as:

   a. Client is experiencing anxiety due to paranoid delusions.
   b. Client will talk with nursing staff 2 times a shift.
   c. Client will be less confused.
   d. Client's self-esteem is impaired.

4. Akathisia is assessed by observing which client response?

   a. Seizure
   b. Muscle spasm
   c. Motor restlessness
   d. Resting tremor

5. When recording objective data regarding client status, the nurse might include which of the following on the client's chart?

   a. Client complains of hearing voices.
   b. Client states that she is angry.
   c. "There are bugs on the wall," shouted Ms. Rodriguez.
   d. Client has a flat affect.

6. The nurse who experiences strong negative feelings toward a new client on the unit should:

   a. Tell the client about these feelings.
   b. Disregard the feelings.
   c. Discuss the feelings with a trusted staff member.
   d. Recognize that negative feelings toward clients are abnormal.

7. Social factors that might contribute to a psychiatric client's illness are best obtained from:

   a. Projective tests.
   b. Genograms.
   c. Intelligence tests.
   d. Previous medical records.

8. Mr. Wright was admitted to a psychiatric unit with a diagnosis of bipolar disorder. He is hyperactive and has not slept or eaten for several days. The nurse should first evaluate Mr. Wright for which needs?

   a. Physiologic needs
   b. Safety and security
   c. Self-esteem
   d. Love and belonging

9. Harold is diagnosed with dysthymia and is at risk for developing major depression. Harold became acutely depressed with suicidal ideation after he lost his job due to reorganization within his firm. Upon his admission to the psychiatric unit, the initial concern of the nursing staff would be to:

   a. Understand the reason for Harold's depression.
   b. Identify Harold's coping skills.
   c. Assess Harold's family support system.
   d. Protect Harold from self-harm.

10. As Harold progresses in treatment, the nurse looks for subjective signs of improvement. Which of the following is a subjective indicator?

    a. Harold begins eating.
    b. Harold talks in group therapy.
    c. Harold says that he feels better.
    d. Harold agrees to take medicine.

1. **Correct answer is b.** Preoccupation with thoughts, avoiding eye contact, and inappropriate laughter are objective indications that the client is hearing voices. The nurse should corroborate this assessment with subjective data by asking the client if he/she is hearing voices.

   a. A phobia is indicated by a severe anxiety reaction to a specific stimulus.
   c. Flight of ideas is indicated when the client's speech jumps from topic to topic.
   d. Loose associations is indicated when the client's speech shows an illogical stream of thought.

2. **Correct answer is c.** The client is able to progress from the concrete image of a "rolling stone" and "moss" to the concepts of stability and friendship.

   a, b, and **d.** These are concrete interpretations of the proverb and contain no abstract concepts.

3. **Correct answer is b.** Plans are measurable, indicate client outcomes, and set specific time frames.

   a. This statement indicates a client assessment, not a plan.
   c. This is a weak plan. It is not measurable and does not indicate a specific time frame.
   d. This statement indicates a client assessment, not a plan.

4. **Correct answer is c.** Akathisia is a side effect of antipsychotic medication and manifests as extreme motor restlessness. Subjectively, the client may complain of the inability to sit still.

   a, b, and **d.** These are not components of akathisia.

5. **Correct answer is d.** Objective data are indicated by what the nurse is able to observe directly.

   a, b, and **c.** These are subjective reports by the client.

6. **Correct answer is c.** The nurse is most likely experiencing negative transference, a projection of feelings from the nurse's past onto the current situation. Self-awareness and analysis of personal feelings are necessary in psychiatric nursing, and feelings are frequently shared with team members.

   a. Although it may be appropriate to share personal reactions in certain situations (e.g., when the client is trying to correct certain behaviors that provoke negative feelings in others), it would not be helpful in this case to share the nurse's personal reaction with the client.
   b. Disregarding feelings may impair the nurse's ability to develop a therapeutic relationship with the client.
   d. As the nurse recognizes that she/he may have many different feelings, the ability to accept the client's feelings is enhanced.

7. **Correct answer is b.** Genograms demonstrate past and present family constellations and patterns of events that affect an individual's social well-being.

   a. Projective tests are useful to evaluate personality traits.
   c. Intelligence tests are useful to evaluate for the presence and degree of mental retardation.
   d. Although it is useful to consult the client's medical history, changes may have occurred in the client's social system since the last treatment.

8. **Correct answer is a.** According to Maslow's human needs theory, unmet needs constitute a problem. Client is likely to be dehydrated due to hyperactivity and reduced calorie and fluid intake. Physiologic needs are the priority in the hierarchy of needs.

   b. Safety and security needs are significant in a hyperactive client but do not surpass the physiologic needs in this case. Safety and security needs are a priority when the client is a danger to self or others.

c. Self-esteem may be a concern for this client, but not during the acute phase of the illness. When the client's mental status improves and he begins to think about the future, relationships, and success, self-esteem needs will then be addressed.

d. Love and belonging may be a concern for this client, but not during the acute phase of the illness. When the client is able to look at developing relationships, then love and belonging needs will become a priority.

9. **Correct answer is d.** When a client demonstrates suicidal ideation, the initial concern of the nursing staff is to ensure a safe environment to protect the patient from self-harm.

a. Depressed clients have difficulty understanding and verbalizing the cause of their illness. It would not be therapeutic to focus on this initially.

b. Harold's coping skills have been compromised, as evidenced by his illness. These may be evaluated as the patient improves.

c. Harold's family support system may become an area of concern when discharge plans are being made.

10. **Correct answer is c.** Client reports his interpretation of an inner state. This personal reflection constitutes a subjective indicator.

a, b, and **d.** These are objective indicators of improvement.

5

Anxiety and Related Disorders

NURSING HIGHLIGHTS

1. Anxiety causes discomfort or distress, which is relieved through a variety of coping mechanisms.
2. Anxiety is communicated between people (e.g., a client who is anxious will trigger feelings of anxiety in a caregiver).
3. Maladaptive, destructive ways of dealing with anxiety may lead to crises, anxiety disorders, pathologic behaviors, or psychotic disorders.
4. Anxiety may be difficult to recognize and diagnose because it is usually accompanied by other emotions and behaviors.

5. Anxiety disorders are characterized by anxiety levels that prevent client from functioning adequately.
6. Cornerstones of treatment for anxiety disorders are (1) to reduce severe levels of anxiety to mild or moderate levels and (2) to teach client effective coping skills.
7. Anxiety levels are reduced through the use of antianxiety medications and nursing interventions that promote relaxation and feelings of calmness and security.
8. Nurse plays a key role in teaching and reinforcing effective coping skills for clients with anxiety disorders.

GLOSSARY

circumstantiality—pattern of speech in which client gives irrelevant details before stating main point

coping mechanisms—conscious or unconscious adaptations in behavior that lower tension in stressful situations

hypervigilance—state of increased alertness, especially in the face of perceived danger

insight therapy—type of psychotherapy in which client is brought to understand the origins of her/his maladaptive behaviors and attitudes

malingering—conscious faking of the symptoms of illness to avoid a situation or to obtain financial gain; distinguished from somatoform disorders, which are involuntary

perceptual field—total environment perceived by an individual at any one time; range of sensory input processed by the brain

primary gain—reduction in anxiety through expression of physical symptoms

psychogenic disorder—any condition resulting from psychologic, mental, or emotional causes

psychophysiologic disorder—any condition that has a physical and a psychologic aspect

psychosomatic disorder—any condition in which physical symptoms are caused by psychologic factors and exist without organic impairment

secondary gain—benefit in addition to reduction in anxiety brought about by expression of symptoms of physical illness

somatization—expression of psychologic stress through physical symptoms

ENHANCED OUTLINE

I. General concepts

A. Anxiety versus fear
   1. Anxiety has no specific object; it is a diffuse sense of uncertainty or apprehension.
   2. Fear has a specific source or object (i.e., one is afraid of something in particular).

See text pages
_____

B. Causes of anxiety: stressors that threaten oneself, one's identity, one's self-esteem, or one's integrated social functioning; may be real or perceived
   1. Fear of punishment, disapproval, threatened withdrawal of love, physical harm, etc.
   2. Anticipated loss of bodily control (e.g., in a client facing a degenerative disease)
   3. Anticipated loss of freedom, self-determination
   4. Anticipated isolation—loss of relationships

C. Responses to anxiety
   1. Fight-or-flight response
      a) The fight-or-flight response is a basic response found in many animals as well as humans.
      b) It serves an evolutionary purpose by helping organisms respond to perceived threats.

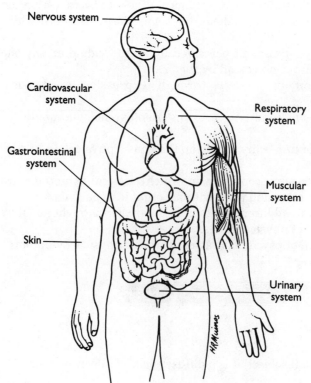

Figure 5–1
Body Systems Affected by Anxiety

c) It causes physiologic and perceptual changes that prepare an organism to fight a potential threat or to flee from it (e.g., increased muscular stimulation, rerouting of blood supply, changes in perceptual field, increased alertness).

d) In humans, a variety of nonphysical threats (such as threat to self-esteem) also trigger the response; when physical fight or flight is impossible or inappropriate, feelings of anxiety result.

2. Physiologic responses (from stimulation of autonomic nervous system)
   a) Cardiovascular responses
      (1) Palpitations
      (2) Increased or decreased pulse rate
      (3) Elevated or lowered blood pressure
      (4) Faintness (syncope)
   b) Respiratory responses
      (1) Rapid breathing
      (2) Shortness of breath
      (3) Feelings of pressure or tightness in the chest
      (4) Feelings of constriction in the throat
      (5) Choking, gasping
      (6) Hyperventilation
   c) Neuromuscular responses
      (1) Heightened reflex response
      (2) Startle reaction
      (3) Tics and twitches
      (4) Insomnia
      (5) Rigidity
      (6) Restlessness
      (7) Pacing
      (8) Generalized weakness
      (9) Shaky knees
    (10) Clumsiness
   d) Gastrointestinal responses
      (1) Loss of appetite
      (2) Abdominal pain or discomfort
      (3) Nausea
      (4) Heartburn
      (5) Diarrhea
   e) Urinary tract responses
      (1) Pressure to urinate
      (2) Frequent urination
   f) Skin responses
      (1) Flushing
      (2) Sweating palms
      (3) Generalized diaphoresis (sweating)
      (4) Itching
      (5) Hives
      (6) Hot or cold flashes
      (7) Pallor, clammy skin

3. Observable behavioral (psychomotor) responses
   a) Restlessness
   b) Physical tension
   c) Rapid speech
   d) Interpersonal withdrawal
   e) Accident-proneness
   f) Inhibition
   g) Flight
   h) Avoidance behaviors
4. Observable cognitive responses
   a) Impaired attention
   b) Impaired concentration
   c) Forgetfulness
   d) Judgment errors
   e) Impaired learning ability
   f) Impaired logic
   g) Impaired reasoning abilities
   h) Preoccupation
   i) Blocking of thoughts
   j) Changes in perceptual field
   k) Diminished productivity and problem-solving abilities and reduced creativity
   l) Confusion
   m) Hypervigilance
   n) Self-consciousness
   o) Lack of perspective, objectivity
   p) Loss of control, fear of losing control
5. Observable affective responses
   a) Edginess
   b) Impatience
   c) Uneasiness
   d) Fearfulness
   e) Nervous tension
   f) Jumpiness
   g) Alarm
   h) Terror

D. Anxiety continuums
   1. Continuum of severity
      a) Mild anxiety
         (1) Associated with day-to-day living
         (2) Increases alertness
         (3) Enlarges a person's perceptual field
         (4) Can motivate learning and creativity

b) Moderate anxiety
   (1) Focuses attention on immediate concerns
   (2) Narrows perceptual field, blocking out selected areas
c) Severe anxiety
   (1) Narrows perceptual field even further
   (2) Focuses attention on a specific detail, causing person to lose sight of the larger picture
   (3) Behavior directed at relieving anxiety
d) Panic
   (1) Complete loss of perspective
   (2) Overwhelming sensations of terror, dread, awe
   (3) Increased motor activity
   (4) Severe disturbances in rational thought processes, communication, function
   (5) Disorganization of personality
   (6) Can be life-threatening
2. Adaptive-maladaptive and constructive-destructive continuums
   a) Mild and moderate levels of anxiety can be a positive force; they provide an impetus for initiating or changing behavior (e.g., anxiety over one's performance on an upcoming examination provides a stimulus to engage in anxiety-reducing behavior [i.e., studying for the exam]).
   b) Anxiety disorders occur when anxiety impairs normal functioning. Psychiatric problems may arise when anxiety levels are overwhelming (e.g., as a result of physical trauma) or because the client uses relatively ineffective coping mechanisms.
   c) Excessive or unresolved anxiety may be expressed in a variety of ways, such as panic, obsessions, compulsions, phobias.

E. Coping mechanisms to relieve anxiety: may be adaptive or maladaptive, constructive or destructive; may be employed with or without conscious thought
   1. Acting-out behaviors (intense expressions of feeling)
      a) Behaviors originating on unconscious level to relieve anxiety and tension
      b) Examples: anger, crying, laughter, physical exertion, cursing
   2. Somatizing
      a) Experience of psychic stress as a physical reaction
      b) Examples: headache, backache, stomach pains
   3. Avoidance (e.g., lack of eye contact, superficiality, daydreaming)
   4. Problem solving: talking it out, thinking it through
   5. Task-oriented responses: usually used by individuals experiencing moderate, severe, or panic levels of anxiety
      a) Attack: deliberate action to confront or resolve anxiety source; may be constructive or destructive
      b) Withdrawal: action to remove oneself from the anxiety-provoking situation; may be constructive or destructive
         (1) Physical withdrawal (e.g., removing oneself from a smoke-filled room, dropping a class)
         (2) Psychologic withdrawal (e.g., apathy, admitting defeat, isolation)

       c) Compromise: a usually constructive action to mitigate the potential negative effects of anxiety; an appropriate response when attack and withdrawal are not possible or effective; used to change one's usual way of responding

6. Defense mechanisms (also called ego-oriented reactions)
   a) Behaviors operating on a relatively unconscious level
   b) Used by everyone to protect the self from feelings of inadequacy and loss of self-esteem
   c) May be adaptive (healthy) or maladaptive (unhealthy) (i.e., may help one cope with anxiety in constructive or destructive manner)
      (1) Adaptive uses allow individual to function personally and socially during times of anxiety.
      (2) Maladaptive uses do not effectively reduce anxiety and may cause interference with personal, work, and social goals; they include inappropriate frequency, intensity, and duration of defense mechanism.
   d) May be any of several types
      (1) Compensation: making up for a perceived failing by emphasizing another quality or asset (e.g., emphasizing one's intellect to compensate for failed social relationships)
      (2) Denial: ignoring or refusing to acknowledge painful or negative facts (e.g., A mother does not believe the doctor's diagnosis that her child has cancer.)
      (3) Displacement: shifting emotions to a "safe" alternative (e.g., A child who is angry at a parent hits a younger sibling.)
      (4) Dissociation: separating a group of mental and/or behavioral processes from one's consciousness (e.g., getting amnesia after a traumatic event)
      (5) Identification: attempting to become like an admired person by taking on his/her opinions, mannerisms, behavior, etc.
      (6) Introjection: an intense form of identification, often seen in toddlers as part of normal development (e.g., A young boy dresses like an admired sports figure.)
      (7) Intellectualization: excessive use of logic or reasoning to avoid anxiety-provoking thoughts or conclusions (e.g., A client masks fear of public places by creating logical reasons for avoiding them—they're crowded, they're unsafe, etc.)
      (8) Isolation: separating emotional content from a thought (e.g., a woman who shows no emotion when discussing her abusive spouse)
      (9) Projection: projecting one's thoughts or emotions onto another person (e.g., A person who feels insecure accuses his/her spouse of feeling insecure.)

(10) Rationalization: fixing blame for a perceived failing on someone or something other than the self by offering a socially acceptable, plausible reason for the behavior (e.g., A student who receives a poor grade says that the instructor was poor.)

(11) Reaction formation: development of conscious thoughts and emotions that are the opposite of one's true feelings or desires (e.g., One who is afraid of another treats him/her with contempt or hostility.)

(12) Regression: a retreat to an earlier developmental stage as a reaction to anxiety (e.g., A child may begin sucking his/her thumb upon the birth of a sibling.)

(13) Repression: unconscious exclusion of painful thoughts from the consciousness (e.g., forgetting a doctor's appointment because of fear of a poor diagnosis)

(14) Suppression: conscious exclusion of painful thoughts (e.g., putting off making a doctor's appointment in the face of symptoms of illness)

(15) Splitting: looking upon people, self, or situations as being all good or all bad

(16) Sublimation: substituting a socially acceptable goal for a goal that is unattainable or blocked (e.g., channeling one's aggression into one's work)

(17) Undoing: committing an act that symbolically or actually negates a prior one (e.g., Two people engage in small talk after an emotionally charged confrontation.)

F. Theoretic explanations of anxiety disorders
  1. Psychodynamic theory
     a) It is based on psychoanalytic theory.
     b) It assumes that anxiety is a signal to the ego to take defensive action.
     c) Freud identified the source of anxiety as intrapsychic conflicts (i.e., forbidden sexual or aggressive impulses that must be repressed).
     d) Sullivan identified the source of anxiety as interpersonal conflicts, beginning with one's first experiences in infancy.
  2. Behavioral theory
     a) Behavioral techniques have proven to be effective treatments for phobias and obsessive-compulsive disorder, suggesting that at least some types of anxiety are a learned response.
     b) Behavioral theory assumes that anxiety develops as a conditioned response to certain stimuli.
  3. Biologic theory
     a) Evidence suggests that in some cases anxiety may be due to physiologic abnormalities (e.g., obesity).
     b) The effectiveness of antianxiety medications is evidence of a physical basis, at least in part, for anxiety disorders.

I. General concepts	II. Treatments for anxiety disorders	III. Essential nursing care for anxiety	IV. Specific anxiety disorders	V. Somatoform disorders

See text pages

II. Treatments for anxiety disorders (may be used singly or in combination)

A. Antianxiety medications (short-term use) (see Nurse Alert, "Antianxiety Medications: Risks and Cautions")
   1. Benzodiazepines
   2. Propranediols
   3. Acetylinic alcohol
   4. Diphenylmethane antihistamines

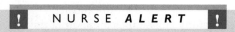

! NURSE *ALERT* !

Antianxiety Medications: Risks and Cautions

- **benzodiazepines:** Useful for short-term treatment during a time of specific stress. Minimal potential for overdose when used alone; however, may cause lethal overdose when combined with alcohol. Often cause drowsiness. High risk for dependence with long-term use. Withdrawal symptoms (e.g., dizziness, irritability) if discontinued too quickly. Should not be used during pregnancy. Examples: diazepam (Valium), chlordiazepoxide (Librium)

- **propranediols:** Sedative-hypnotic drugs with antianxiety effects. High risk for tolerance and addiction, creating risks of withdrawal symptoms including insomnia, anxiety, hallucinations, and seizures. High risk for overdose. Often cause drowsiness, depression of central nervous system (CNS). Rarely used because of high risk for addiction and availability of more effective drugs. Example: meprobamate (Equanil)

- **acetylinic alcohol:** A sedative-hypnotic drug with antianxiety effects; risks are similar to those of propranediols. May cause confusion, ataxia, hypotension, exaggerated depression with deep sleep and muscle weakness. Example: ethchlorvynol (Placidyl)

- **diphenylmethane antihistamines:** Do not cause physical dependence or abuse. Minimal toxicity. Generally safe for long-term use. Less effective than benzodiazepines. May cause drowsiness. Have aftertaste. Example: hydroxyzine HCL (Atarax)

- **buspirone hydrochloride (Buspar):** New drug; causes less sedation than benzodiazepines. Does not seem to cause dependence. Delayed onset of effects for up to 3 weeks. Does not interact with CNS depressants.

- **beta-adrenergic blocker:** Primarily used as a heart medication; it blocks the effects of the autonomic nervous system and thereby relieves physical symptoms of anxiety such as tachycardia. Often prescribed for stage fright. No potential for dependence or abuse. Risk for hypotension, bradycardia. Example: propranolol (Inderal)

- **tricyclic antidepressants:** Help prevent panic attacks by regulating brain's supply of serotonin. Used for severe obsessive-compulsive disorder. Delayed onset of action. Very limited potential for dependence or abuse. Should not be stopped suddenly. May cause seizures, cardiac arrhythmias. May cause dry mouth, grogginess, weight gain, blurred vision, constipation. Examples: clomipramine (Anafranil), imipramine (Tofranil)

5. Buspirone hydrochloride
6. Beta-adrenergic blocker
7. Tricyclic antidepressants

B. Psychotherapy
   1. Behavior modification
      a) Systematic desensitization: combining deep muscle relaxation with exposure to a series of encounters with an anxiety-provoking stimulus, beginning with the least frightening and progressing to the most frightening
      b) Biofeedback: the use of electronic sensors and monitors to help client develop stress-reduction techniques and control over autonomic functions
   2. Cognitive therapy
   3. Transactional analysis
   4. Family therapy
   5. Group therapy
   6. Psychoanalysis

C. Health teaching methods for handling stress: techniques that introduce the relaxation response in the body (see Client Teaching Checklist, "Initiating the Relaxation Response")
   1. Meditation: technique in which the client focuses on a mantra (image or word that is chanted aloud) to achieve an altered state of consciousness
   2. Visualization: use of an in-depth mental picture of a relaxing, pleasant situation or scene; can be used with other relaxation techniques
   3. Physical exercise
   4. Progressive muscular relaxation (PMR): deep muscle relaxation achieved through tensing and releasing muscles or muscle groups 1 at a time (active PMR) or through consciously relaxing muscles without first tensing them (passive PMR)

III. Essential nursing care for anxiety

See text pages
_____

A. Nursing assessment
   1. Take histories.
      a) Medical
      b) Psychiatric
      c) Family
      d) Social
      e) Of present problem
   2. Assess current mental status: Record observations of client's behavior and affect to determine level of anxiety.
   3. When possible (at mild or moderate anxiety levels), interview client.
      a) Identify precipitating stressor or stressors that caused anxiety.
      b) Identify effect of stress on client's daily life.
   4. Assess responses to anxiety.
      a) Physiologic (same as section I,C,2 of this chapter)
      b) Behavioral (psychomotor) (same as section I,C,3 of this chapter)

      c) Cognitive (same as section I,C,4 of this chapter)

      d) Affective (same as section I,C,5 of this chapter)

   5. Assess coping mechanisms.

      a) Identify constructive and destructive coping mechanisms.

      b) Assess appropriateness of coping mechanisms to perceived threat.

   6. Differentiate anxiety responses from other psychiatric conditions.

      a) Anxiety versus psychosis: Anxiety responses usually do not involve distortion of reality, though psychosis (distortion of reality) may occur with panic levels of anxiety.

      b) Anxiety versus depression

         (1) Anxiety and depression often coexist, share similar symptoms (e.g., sleep disturbances, appetite changes, fatigue, helplessness).

         (2) Depression generally involves more global feelings of despair, hopelessness, and sadness.

✔ CLIENT TEACHING CHECKLIST ✔

Initiating the Relaxation Response

The relaxation response is the counterpoint to the fight-or-flight response. It reduces the physical responses of the sympathetic nervous system that prepare the body to react to stress by fighting or fleeing. It is the action of the parasympathetic nervous system that reduces the body's heart rate, breathing rate, metabolism, blood pressure, and muscular tension. By relieving the physical responses associated with anxiety, the relaxation response promotes clear, calm thinking and helps the client implement other healthy coping responses. Each type of relaxation therapy uses techniques that produce the relaxation response.

Typical relaxation procedures include the following instructions:

✔ Choose a quiet area where you will not be interrupted. Dim the lights if you wish.

✔ Choose a comfortable position.

✔ Breathe in a rhythmic pattern. Breathe in deeply; exhale slowly.

✔ Select a word or visualize a scene that promotes relaxation and that can serve as a focus for concentration.

✔ Push distractions aside gently. If they enter the mind, have a passive attitude. Do not worry about them. Do not try too hard to relax.

✔ Close your eyes.

✔ (Nurse may wish to introduce elements of progressive muscular relaxation here.) Do a body scanning (i.e., identify muscles that are particularly tense [often the muscles of the back, neck, and face]). Tighten, then release 1 group of muscles at a time (e.g., the left hand, then the right hand).

✔ During the exercise, focus on the chosen word or scene to prevent distractions from entering the mind.

✔ Repeat the procedure once or twice a day for 20–30 minutes each time.

7. Differentiate anxiety responses from mimickers (i.e., physical disorders that produce symptoms resembling anxiety or panic attacks, such as Ménière's syndrome, mitral valve prolapse, uncontrolled diabetes).
8. Assess potential for harm to client or others.

B. Nursing diagnoses
   1. Main NANDA nursing diagnoses
      a) Anxiety
      b) Ineffective individual coping
      c) Fear
   2. Additional NANDA nursing diagnoses
      a) Impaired adjustment
      b) Impaired verbal communication
      c) Altered thought processes
      d) Self-esteem disturbance
      e) Potential for injury
      f) Risk for trauma
      g) Posttrauma response
      h) Powerlessness
      i) Altered role performance
      j) Impaired social interaction
      k) Social isolation
      l) Self-care deficits
      m) Ineffective breathing pattern
      n) Altered sensory perceptions
      o) Altered nutrition
      p) Sleep pattern disturbance
      q) Impaired skin integrity
      r) Diarrhea
      s) Altered urinary elimination
   3. Selected complete nursing diagnoses
      a) Panic level of anxiety related to family rejection evidenced by confusion and impaired judgment
      b) Moderate anxiety related to financial pressures evidenced by inhibition and avoidance
      c) Ineffective individual coping related to academic performance evidenced by psychomotor disturbances
      d) Fear related to abuse evidenced by agitation and abdominal pain

C. Planning (goal setting)
   1. General goals
      a) Help client identify feelings as anxiety.
      b) Reduce level of severe anxiety/panic through nursing interventions that support and protect client.
      c) Help client with mild/moderate anxiety first to not increase level of anxiety and then to decrease level.
      d) Help client develop ability to cope with mild anxiety and use it constructively.

2. Examples of specific goals
   a) Client will identify feelings as anxiety.
   b) Client will verbalize feeling less anxious.
   c) Physical symptoms of anxiety will be diminished (e.g., pulse rate will decrease to normal, diaphoresis will resolve).
   d) Client with a phobia will be able to tolerate exposure to the object of his/her phobia.
   e) Client with compulsive disorder will exhibit decreased frequency of ritualistic behaviors.
   f) Client with obsessive disorder will verbalize fewer obsessive statements.
   g) Client will achieve satisfactory role performance (e.g., will attend school or work daily, will resume normal family obligations).

D. Nursing implementation (intervention)
   1. General interventions for all levels of anxiety
      a) Help client feel secure and accepted without encouraging dependency.
         (1) Listen to client.
         (2) Employ empathy.
      b) Help client identify feelings as anxiety.
      c) Assist client in understanding precipitators of his/her anxiety.
         (1) Encourage client to describe his/her feelings.
         (2) Help client see links between his/her feelings and behavior.
         (3) Educate client on mechanisms, causes, and physical effects of anxiety.
      d) Assist client in identifying and developing adaptive coping mechanisms and healthy behavior.
         (1) Explore acts and behaviors that have helped relieve anxiety in the past (see Client Teaching Checklist, "Helping Clients Identify Effective Coping Strategies").
         (2) Offer positive reinforcement for healthy behavior.
      e) Support client as she/he develops new coping mechanisms.
         (1) Help client practice stress-reducing relaxation techniques.
         (2) Offer positive feedback.
      f) Assist client in relating new knowledge to his/her life situation.
         (1) Help client tolerate mild anxiety and use it constructively.
         (2) Provide opportunities for normal, healthy interaction and role behaviors.
         (3) Rehearse potentially stressful situations.
      g) Assist client's family in changing dysfunctional or maladaptive behavioral patterns.
         (1) Teach family members to reinforce client's healthy behaviors.
         (2) Teach family not to "protect" client by taking over his/her normal functions or roles.

Helping Clients Identify Effective Coping Strategies

Clients with anxiety disorders usually lack insight into the effects of the coping strategies they use. In addition, they have not identified alternative coping strategies that would be more effective in reducing anxiety. The following questions can help the client assess and analyze coping mechanisms used in the past and can help identify new strategies for dealing with anxiety:

✔ What events can you think of that might have caused these anxiety reactions? (If the client cannot name any, you can rephrase the question: Tell me about some of the things that were going on in your life just before you came in for help.)

✔ How did you feel when these events occurred?

✔ What did you do about those feelings? Did you try to make them stop? How?

✔ Were you successful in making the feelings go away?

✔ Did the feelings come back later? What did you do about them?

✔ Can you name other ways you might have dealt with those feelings?

✔ Do you think some ways are better than others? Why?

✔ How do you know when you're upset or tense? Some people, for example, feel a knot in their stomach or get a headache, or they can't concentrate.

✔ When these signs occur, what do you usually do? Does it work?

✔ What else could you do that might work better?

✔ What are the most common things that make you upset or tense? Many people, for example, get tense when they're late for an appointment.

✔ What can you do to change or eliminate the things that make you tense or upset?

   (3) Teach family to give attention to client, not symptoms.
   (4) Explore family's underlying and unresolved anxiety-provoking issues and coping patterns; teach effective coping techniques to family.
2. Interventions for severe and panic levels of anxiety
   a) Relieve immediate distress.
      (1) Stay with client.
      (2) Acknowledge anxiety.
      (3) Speak slowly and calmly.
      (4) Use short words and sentences; repeat if necessary.
      (5) Project sense of confidence and control, that you can help and protect client.
      (6) Help direct client's behavior.
      (7) Decrease excessive stimuli and stressful interactions.
      (8) Walk with client who is pacing.
      (9) Increase supervision for acutely anxious clients, to prevent harm to self and/or loss of control; speak firmly when setting physical limits.
      (10) Do not challenge client's defense mechanisms unless his/her physical well-being is threatened; challenging defenses in acute anxiety increases anxiety and may cause panic.

        (11) Administer antianxiety medications as ordered; observe for side effects.

    b) Develop therapeutic relationship of trust.

    c) Assess and control own feelings, to avoid increasing client's anxiety levels.

      (1) Respect and protect client's comfort level; implement active interventions, such as insight therapy, only as the client begins to feel comfortable.

      (2) Avoid ridicule or expressing value judgments regarding coping mechanisms, even those that are maladaptive.

    d) Promote physical activity to discharge client's anxiety.

    e) Promote tissue perfusion and elimination, as increased activity of autonomic nervous system may cause circulatory and digestive system disturbances.

    f) Promote personal hygiene and grooming: assess skin integrity, hygienic practices; provide assistance and health teaching as required.

  3. Interventions for moderate levels of anxiety

    a) Offer acceptance and support.

    b) Establish trust.

    c) Promote communication.

    d) Concentrate on the client's concerns.

    e) Help client identify his/her anxiety and its precipitating stressors.

      (1) Use questions (e.g., "Are you uncomfortable?").

      (2) Relate behavior to anxiety (e.g., when a client is tapping a foot, ask, "Are you feeling anxious now?").

      (3) Overcome resistance (e.g., denial, rationalization).

    f) Implement stress-reducing techniques, such as deep breathing, visualization, massage, meditation, progressive relaxation.

    g) Encourage client to use coping mechanisms that have proved successful in the past and to avoid those that were unsuccessful or harmful.

    h) To encourage client to try new coping mechanisms, use role-playing techniques and feedback to reinforce them.

    i) Allow time for client to practice and integrate new coping techniques.

    j) Offer positive reinforcement for healthy behaviors.

    k) Help client identify ways to restructure goals or modify behavior.

    l) Focus responsibility for change on client.

E. Nursing evaluation

  1. Evaluation of goal achievement is ongoing; goals and care plan are revised as needed.

    a) Client's panic/severe level of anxiety is reduced to moderate level.

    b) Client with mild/moderate anxiety does not increase anxiety level and is able to decrease level.

     c) Client is able to use mild anxiety constructively.

     d) Client gained insights into causes of anxiety and can identify own response to anxiety.

     e) Client reduced maladaptive responses and developed constructive coping mechanisms.

     f) Client achieved satisfactory role performance.

  2. If goals were not achieved, assess reasons.

     a) Were goals realistic?

     b) Were problems identified correctly?

     c) Was enough time allowed for achievement of goals?

IV. Specific anxiety disorders (DSM-IV)

(For all anxiety disorders in this section, refer to section III of this chapter for essential nursing care; where appropriate, specific nursing interventions are described for a particular disorder.)

> See text pages
> _____

A. Generalized anxiety disorder

  1. Definition: excessive anxiety and worry, occurring more days than not for at least 6 months, about a number of events or activities, in the absence of phobias, panic attacks, obsessive-compulsive disorder, separation anxiety disorder, and posttraumatic stress disorder

  2. At least 3 of the following 6 symptoms:

     a) Restlessness, edginess

     b) Easily tired

     c) Difficulty concentrating

     d) Irritability

     e) Muscle tension

     f) Sleeping difficulty (inability to sleep, disturbances during sleep)

  3. Treatments (may be used singly or in combination)

     a) Antianxiety medications (short-term use)

     b) Psychotherapy

     c) Relaxation therapy

B. Panic disorder (with or without agoraphobia)

  1. Definition: recurrent unexpected panic attacks with discrete period of intense fear or discomfort

  2. At least 4 of the following symptoms, which develop abruptly and peak within 10 minutes:

     a) Dyspnea (shortness of breath)

     b) Palpitations or tachycardia

     c) Chest discomfort or pain

     d) Feeling of choking

     e) Dizziness

     f) Abdominal distress or nausea

     g) Diaphoresis (sweating)

     h) Hot or cold flashes

     i) Trembling or shaking

     j) Paresthesias (tingling of hands or feet)

     k) Feelings of unreality (derealization)

l) Fear of losing control

m) Fear of dying

3. Treatments (may be used singly or in combination)

a) Imipramine (to prevent panic attacks)

b) Psychotherapy

c) Relaxation therapy

C. Obsessive-compulsive disorder

1. Definition

a) Obsession: preoccupation with persistent, intrusive thoughts, impulses, or images that client cannot dismiss

b) Compulsion: repetitive, purposeful performance of anxiety-reducing rituals over which client feels he/she has no control

2. Main types

a) Obsessions: rigid thoughts related to:

(1) Dirt, germs

(2) Aggression

(3) Orderliness

(4) Sexual behavior

(5) Religion

b) Compulsions

(1) Excessive washing

(2) Checking certain objects

c) May be combined

3. Treatments (may be used singly or in combination)

a) Antianxiety medications (short-term use) (e.g., clomipramine)

b) Behavior modification

c) Cognitive therapy

d) Family therapy

e) Psychotherapy

f) Relaxation therapy

4. Nursing interventions

a) Reduce anxiety and need for rituals (e.g., administer medications on time, provide explanations before a procedure or activity, don't keep client waiting for appointments).

b) Don't interfere with rituals initially.

c) Provide time for rituals.

d) Remain nonjudgmental and protect client from ridicule of others.

e) Gradually reduce time available for rituals as client becomes involved in other activities (i.e., gradually substitute healthy behaviors for rituals).

f) Help client identify anxiety-causing situations that lead to ritualistic behavior.

g) Teach client how to interrupt ritual patterns.

h) Help client speak simply, to reduce circumstantiality.

i) Offer support; let client know that mistakes are permitted.

j) Give client positive reinforcement for adaptive, nonritualistic behaviors.

D. Phobias

1. Definition: fears that the client acknowledges as irrational but that persist nonetheless

2. Types

a) Agoraphobia without history of panic disorder: anxiety about being in places or situations from which escape might be difficult or embarrassing or in which help may not be available

b) Specific phobia: marked, persistent fear, set off by the presence or anticipation of a specific object or situation (e.g., flying, high places, enclosed places)

c) Social phobia (social anxiety disorder): marked, persistent fear of 1 or more social or performance situations

3. Treatments (may be used singly or in combination)

a) Behavior modification: to weaken bond between stimulus and response

   (1) Systematic desensitization (see section II,B,1,a of this chapter)

   (2) Reciprocal inhibition: pairing of anxiety-provoking stimulus with an anxiety-relieving stimulus (such as biofeedback) to reduce maladaptive response to anxiety-provoking stimulus

   (3) Exposure (flooding): repeated contact with anxiety-provoking stimuli until anxiety diminishes (use is controversial, as it may exacerbate anxiety responses)

   (4) Cognitive restructuring (relabeling): changing how a situation is experienced by relabeling it (e.g., by labeling an anxiety-provoking situation as exciting or challenging)

b) Antianxiety medications (short-term use)

c) Psychotherapy

d) Cognitive therapy

e) Relaxation therapy

f) Family therapy

g) Propranolol (for stage fright)

4. Nursing interventions

a) Accept client's fears nonjudgmentally.

b) Encourage verbalization of fears.

c) Do not characterize phobias as silly or insignificant, even if the client does; acknowledge and explain that all behavior serves some purpose.

d) Do not force client to confront the object of his/her phobia; panic may result.

e) Promote effective role performance through gradual application of desensitization or other therapies.

E. Posttraumatic stress disorder (PTSD)
   1. Definition: development of characteristic symptoms after unusually stressful events (such as combat, violent crime, abuse, natural disaster)
   2. Types
      a) Acute: duration of symptoms, less than 3 months
      b) Chronic: duration of symptoms, 3 months or more
      c) Delayed onset: appearance of symptoms at least 6 months after trauma
   3. Symptoms
      a) Traumatic event is persistently reexperienced through, for example, distressing dreams, flashbacks, or reliving of the event.
      b) Client persistently avoids stimuli associated with the trauma and exhibits a numbing of general responsiveness.
      c) Client experiences persistent symptoms of increased arousal such as:
         (1) Sleep disturbance
         (2) Anger
         (3) Hypervigilance
         (4) Exaggerated startle response
         (5) Difficulty concentrating
   4. Treatments (may be used singly or in combination)
      a) Antianxiety medications (short-term use)
      b) Crisis intervention (in acute stage)
      c) Family therapy
      d) Psychotherapy
      e) Relaxation therapy
      f) Self-help groups
      g) Desensitization therapy
   5. Nursing interventions
      a) Provide general nursing support.
      b) Encourage expression of feelings.
      c) Refer client for therapy.
      d) Reinforce insights gained through therapy.
      e) Provide appropriate support as client moves through 4 stages of adjustment.
         (1) Recovery: Client realizes that he/she is safe from harm.
         (2) Avoidance: Client tries not to think about experiences in order to avoid overwhelming feelings.
         (3) Reconsideration: Client reflects on past experiences, begins to confront thoughts and feelings.
         (4) Adjustment: Client begins to become reintegrated into his/her environment.

V. Somatoform disorders: conditions in which an individual experiences physical symptoms of illness for which there is no organic or physiologic cause

See text pages
_____

A. General concepts

  1. Somatoform disorders involve the expression of anxiety as physical symptoms, often involving sensory or motor functions.
  2. Physical symptoms are not under voluntary control; client believes symptoms are real.
  3. Somatoform disorders provide primary and secondary gains.
     a) The primary gain, which operates on an unconscious level, is the reduction of anxiety.
     b) Secondary gains are avoidance of anxiety-provoking situations by displaying physical symptoms and positive reinforcement (for example, when illness brings attention or sympathy).

B. Types (DSM-IV)

  1. Somatization disorder
     a) Client presents with multiple, recurrent physical complaints for which medical attention has been sought but for which there is no organic reason.
     b) Onset of symptoms occurs before age 30.
     c) Client experiences symptoms for several years.
     d) Each symptom must not be fully explained by a known medical condition, and the complaints must have caused significant impairment in social or occupational functioning.
  2. Conversion disorder
     a) Client experiences loss or alteration of a physical function suggestive of a physical disorder (e.g., blindness, seizures, paralysis).
     b) The conversion occurs soon after stress.
     c) It occurs without the client's conscious intent.
     d) The physical symptom is symbolically related to psychologic conflict or need (e.g., a man who witnesses a death may go blind).
     e) The symptom or deficit cannot be explained by a neurologic or general medical condition.
     f) The symptom or deficit causes clinically significant distress or impairment in social, occupational, or other aspects of life.
  3. Pain disorder (called somatoform pain disorder in DSM-III-R)
     a) Pain is experienced in 1 or more anatomic sites.
     b) The pain causes clinically significant distress or impairment.
     c) Psychologic factors are important to the onset, severity, worsening, or continuation of the pain.
     d) There are 2 categories of pain disorder.
        (1) Pain disorder associated solely or primarily with psychologic factors
           (a) Disorder is closely associated in time with a stressor.
           (b) Disorder allows the client to avoid something unpleasant.
           (c) Disorder allows the client to obtain support that he/she would not be able to get otherwise (e.g., attention from a spouse or parent).

(2) Pain disorder associated with both psychologic factors and a general medical condition

    4. Hypochondriasis
      a) Client unrealistically interprets minor physical symptoms as indicative of serious illness, leading to preoccupation.
      b) Client's belief that she/he has a serious illness persists despite appropriate medical evaluation and reassurance.
      c) Client's belief causes clinically significant distress or impairment.
      d) The duration is at least 6 months.
    5. Body dysmorphic disorder
      a) Client is preoccupied with an imagined defect in physical appearance or places unwarranted emphasis on a minor physical abnormality or problem.
      b) The preoccupation causes clinically significant distress and impairment.

C. Treatments (may be used singly or in combination)
    1. Behavior modification
    2. Family therapy
    3. Hypnosis/self-hypnosis
    4. Psychotherapy
    5. Relaxation therapy

D. Essential nursing care
    1. Nursing assessment
      a) Take histories.
      b) Record observations of client's behavior and affect.
      c) Assess responses.
      d) Interview client.
        (1) Identify and discuss with client stressful situations that may be the cause of disorder.
        (2) Assess presence of resistance and gaps in information given by client.
        (3) Assess coping mechanisms (e.g., denial, regression, compensation).
      e) Identify constructive versus destructive coping mechanisms.
      f) Record observations to help distinguish from malingering.
      g) Record observations to help distinguish from physical illnesses that have vague or nonspecific symptoms (e.g., mononucleosis, diverticulitis).
        (1) In somatoform disorders, symptoms are often inconsistent with physiology, may change from 1 evaluation to the next, may be subject to suggestions of nurse, physician, or others.

        (2) Client with conversion disorder may exhibit la belle indifférence (lack of concern about symptoms).

        (3) Client with hypochondriasis or somatization disorder may report history of illness and effect of illness on life rather than illness itself.

2. Nursing diagnoses
   a) Main NANDA nursing diagnoses
      (1) Ineffective individual coping
      (2) Impaired adjustment
   b) Additional NANDA nursing diagnoses
      (1) Anxiety
      (2) Ineffective denial
      (3) Altered role performance
      (4) Diversional activity deficit
      (5) Altered family processes
      (6) Fear
      (7) Hopelessness
      (8) Powerlessness
      (9) Self-esteem disturbance
      (10) Social isolation
      (11) Constipation
      (12) Diarrhea
      (13) Impaired gas exchange
      (14) Impaired physical mobility
      (15) Altered nutrition
      (16) Chronic pain
      (17) Self-care deficits
      (18) Impaired skin integrity
      (19) Sleep pattern disturbance
      (20) Body image disturbance
      (21) Altered sensory perceptions
   c) Selected complete nursing diagnoses
      (1) Ineffective individual coping related to impending divorce evidenced by paralysis of right arm
      (2) Social isolation related to chronic pain evidenced by client history

3. Planning (goal setting)
   a) General goals
      (1) Resolve physical symptoms.
      (2) Help client identify underlying anxieties.
      (3) Help client develop healthy coping strategies.
      (4) Eliminate secondary gains.
   b) Examples of specific goals
      (1) Client will no longer experience episodes of severe abdominal pain or will experience them less frequently.
      (2) Client will function appropriately at work and home (e.g., will attend work or school daily, will establish normal social relationships with friends and family).

4. Nursing implementation (intervention)
   a) Maintain the client's biologic integrity by providing for adequate nutrition, hygiene, elimination, and safety needs.
   b) Provide explanations and support during diagnostic tests, to reduce anxiety.
   c) Accept and acknowledge client's perception of symptoms as real; do not imply that symptoms are manufactured or imaginary.
   d) After physical causes have been ruled out, do not reinforce complaints of physical pain or discomfort (e.g., do not take vital signs every time client reports palpitations).
   e) Help client assume responsibility for his/her own physical care, to minimize secondary gain and promote self-esteem.
   f) Observe and record somatic symptoms; notify physician if symptoms persist, to permit evaluation of therapy and to permit reexamination for overlooked physical disease.
   g) Provide full schedule of daily activities, to redirect the client's focus away from physical symptoms and to help relieve underlying anxiety.
   h) Help client focus on emotions rather than on physical symptoms, and encourage client to express his/her feelings about symptoms and their impact on the client's life.
   i) Educate client about how stress and anxiety can produce physical symptoms.
   j) Instruct client in assertiveness techniques to provide an alternative means of getting needs met.
   k) Provide education and support for family regarding causation and need for client to develop and use alternative coping mechanisms.
5. Nursing evaluation
   a) Review goals and assess progress.
      (1) Client becomes less anxious about physical problems.
      (2) Client learns to identify underlying anxieties.
      (3) Client expresses feelings verbally.
      (4) Client reports fewer physical symptoms.
      (5) Client misinterprets reality less often.
      (6) Client is able to go to work and to engage in social activities.
   b) If goals were not achieved, assess reasons.
      (1) Were goals realistic?
      (2) Were problems identified correctly?
      (3) Was enough time allowed for achievement of goals?
      (4) Did the client's circumstances change significantly (e.g., did additional stressors emerge)?
      (5) Were there environmental constraints that prevented achievement of goals?
   c) Revise goals and care plan as necessary.

VI. Dissociative disorders

See text pages

A. General concepts
  1. Dissociative disorders involve the unconscious use of the dissociation defense mechanism, in which anxiety-provoking ideas, emotions, or experiences are separated from one's consciousness and repressed into the unconscious.
  2. Client experiences sudden, temporary inability to integrate her/his identity or motor behavior.
  3. Dissociative disorders provide a means of avoiding anxiety while permitting certain needs to be met.
  4. Forgotten ideas, emotions, or experiences can return to consciousness spontaneously.

B. Types (DSM-IV)
  1. Dissociative amnesia (called psychogenic amnesia in DSM-III-R): 1 or more episodes of inability to recall key information about oneself (information usually of a traumatic or stressful nature); too extensive to be attributed to common forgetfulness
  2. Dissociative fugue (called psychogenic fugue in DSM-III-R)
    a) Client suddenly and unexpectedly travels away from home or from his/her usual workplace and is unable to remember his/her past.
    b) Client is confused about his/her personal identity or assumes a partially or completely new identity.
  3. Dissociative identity disorder (multiple personality disorder)
    a) 2 or more distinct identities or personalities are present in the client.
    b) At least 2 of the identities or personalities recurrently assume control of the client's behavior.
    c) Client can not remember important personal information; inability to recall is too extensive to be attributed to common forgetfulness.
    d) Multiple personality disorder often occurs as a result of childhood physical, emotional, and/or sexual abuse; it is thought to occur when a child is faced with overwhelming and/or repeated anxiety-provoking situations and has not yet formed adequate coping mechanisms.
  4. Depersonalization disorder
    a) Client experiences persistent or recurrent episodes of feeling detached from and as an outside observer of her/his body or thoughts.
    b) During these episodes, client is able to evaluate these situations or experiences objectively and to differentiate between external reality and internal fantasy (reality testing is intact).
    c) The depersonalization causes significant distress or impairment in social, occupational, or other aspects of life.

C. Treatments (often used in combination)
  1. Amytal sodium interview (for multiple personality disorder)
  2. Hypnosis
  3. Psychotherapy
  4. Relaxation therapy

D. Essential nursing care
   1. Nursing assessment
      a) Record observations of client's behavior and affect.
      b) Assess responses.
      c) Assess coping mechanisms.
      d) Perform initial physical examination to differentiate psychogenic amnesia from amnesia related to organic causes (e.g., a head injury).
      e) Take psychosocial history to determine stressful situations that may have contributed to condition.
      f) Identify constructive versus destructive coping mechanisms.
      g) Assess potential for harm to client or others.
   2. Nursing diagnoses
      a) Main NANDA nursing diagnoses
         (1) Ineffective individual coping
         (2) Body image disturbance
         (3) Personal identity disturbance
         (4) Altered role performance
      b) Additional NANDA nursing diagnoses
         (1) Impaired adjustment
         (2) Anxiety
         (3) Altered thought processes
         (4) Self-esteem disturbance
         (5) Impaired verbal communication
         (6) Hopelessness
         (7) Powerlessness
         (8) Potential for injury
         (9) Self-care deficits
         (10) Altered sensory perceptions
         (11) Altered sexuality patterns
         (12) Impaired social interaction
         (13) Social isolation
         (14) High risk for trauma
         (15) Potential for violence, self-directed or directed at others
         (16) Altered family processes
      c) Selected complete nursing diagnoses
         (1) Ineffective individual coping related to history of childhood sexual abuse evidenced by display of multiple personalities
         (2) Altered thought processes related to witnessing a robbery evidenced by inability to recall events before and during the robbery
   3. Planning (setting goals)
      a) General goals
         (1) Provide supportive care.

      (2) Assist client in reintegrating dissociated portions of his/her personality.

      (3) Help client develop effective coping strategies.

  b) Examples of specific goals

      (1) Client will no longer experience symptoms of dissociative disorders or will experience them less frequently.

      (2) Client will resolve underlying anxieties.

      (3) Client will develop healthy coping strategies for anxiety.

      (4) Client will function appropriately at work and home (e.g., will attend work or school daily, will establish normal social relationships with friends and family).

4. Nursing implementation (intervention)

  a) Provide safe, secure environment and frequent monitoring; a sense of estrangement or bewilderment may make the client inattentive to his/her own personal safety.

  b) Establish simple routines for the client, to reduce stress.

  c) Reinforce client's identity and orientation in time and space through frequent use of his/her name, references to date and location, and direct questioning of the client.

  d) Encourage decision making by the client and management of activities of daily living, to promote sense of competence and enhance self-esteem and help keep client grounded in the here-and-now.

  e) Assist in client's decision making as necessary.

  f) Provide support for client's exploration of stressful event(s) that precipitated dissociation episode.

  g) Do not push client to explore too quickly; consequences include provoking anxiety, exacerbating the dissociative episode, and creating resistance.

  h) Help client understand the negative consequences of dissociation.

  i) Help client establish effective coping mechanisms.

  j) Reestablish relationships between client and his/her significant others, if client does not remember these relationships.

5. Nursing evaluation

  a) Review goals and assess progress.

      (1) Client experiences memory loss, disorientation, or altered state of consciousness less frequently.

      (2) Client is able to verbalize feelings about stressful event.

      (3) Client is able to resume social interaction with family and go to work or school.

      (4) Client is able to implement adaptive coping mechanisms.

  b) If goals were not achieved, assess reasons.

      (1) Were goals realistic?

      (2) Were problems identified correctly?

      (3) Was enough time allowed for achievement of goals?

      (4) Did the client's circumstances change significantly (e.g., did additional stressors emerge)?

      (5) Did environmental constraints prevent achievement of goals?

  c) Revise goals and care plan as necessary.

1. Ms. Castro has just been admitted to the nursing unit with a severe level of anxiety. The nurse's initial action should be to:

   a. Stay with Ms. Castro and speak in short, simple sentences.

   b. Have Ms. Castro remain alone in her room until she has better control.

   c. Ask Ms. Castro to describe what is making her so upset.

   d. Explore with Ms. Castro coping mechanisms that have been helpful to her in the past.

2. Alprazolam (Xanax) 1.5 mg BID has been prescribed for Ms. Adams, who has been diagnosed with generalized anxiety disorder. Which statement by Ms. Adams indicates that she understands the role of this medication?

   a. "I plan to treat myself to beer and pizza at least once a week."

   b. "I will take this medicine twice a day while I continue to practice my relaxation techniques."

   c. "After I have several cups of coffee in the morning, I do not feel sleepy from the drug."

   d. "I must never eat within 1 hour of taking the drug."

3. The nurse is assessing Mr. Dalton, who has just been admitted to the nursing unit with a diagnosis of panic disorder. Which statement, if made by Mr. Dalton, would be most consistent with that disorder?

   a. "Sometimes I hear God talking to me through the trees."

   b. "I have not slept in 4 days because I have so many pending business deals that depend on my expertise."

   c. "All of a sudden my heart was pounding, and I was dizzy and couldn't breathe."

   d. "I have been sickly all my life; I must have a heart condition."

4. Ms. Ferrante has been admitted to the nursing unit with a medical diagnosis of obsessive-compulsive disorder. Which of the following statements by Ms. Ferrante best supports a nursing diagnosis of self-esteem disturbance?

   a. "I cannot do things as well as most of the other members of my family."

   b. "I am very shy, and I do not belong to any social groups."

   c. "I wash my hands a lot, and that seems to help when I worry."

   d. "My husband gets angry if I do anything except cook and clean."

5. Which nursing action should take priority early in Ms. Ferrante's hospitalization?

   a. Help Ms. Ferrante verbalize positive aspects of her personality.

   b. Insist that the client attend group functions on the unit.

   c. Provide opportunities for the client to wash her hands when she wishes.

   d. Encourage Mr. and Ms. Ferrante to enter joint counseling.

6. Mr. Harris, who is a student in law school, seeks help for his social phobia, which causes him to fear speaking in public. Which approach by the nurse would be most helpful?

   a. Explain the importance of public speaking to a successful career as a lawyer.

   b. Suggest that Mr. Harris consider a career that does not require speaking in public.

   c. Teach Mr. Harris to use relaxation techniques while he imagines speaking to groups of increasing size.

   d. Call on Mr. Harris to speak unexpectedly to avoid giving him an opportunity to develop anticipatory anxiety.

7. Mr. Jankowicz, a veteran of the Vietnam War, has been hospitalized with symptoms of depression, nightmares, suicidal thinking, anger, and hopelessness. He has experienced

marital discord, alcohol abuse, and inability to hold a job. The nurse would expect which of the following medical diagnoses?

a. Posttraumatic stress disorder
b. Agoraphobia
c. Conversion disorder
d. Dissociative disorder

8. Which nursing diagnosis should have the highest priority early in Mr. Jankowicz's hospitalization?

a. Knowledge deficit
b. Ineffective individual coping
c. Social isolation
d. Potential for violence

9. Mr. Jankowicz will experience the most lasting relief of his symptoms when he is able to:

a. Comply with the prescribed medication program.
b. Receive more sympathetic support from his wife and family.
c. Discuss his sad and bitter memories with sympathetic listeners.
d. Understand the negative effects of alcohol on his body.

10. Ms. Kalen comes to the nursing unit with a provisional diagnosis of somatization disorder. The nurse's initial focus for care would be:

a. Overcoming Ms. Kalen's reluctance to discuss her history of physical symptoms.
b. Insisting that Ms. Kalen participate in unit activities, even when she feels ill.
c. Evaluating Ms. Kalen to be certain that no physical illness exists.
d. Explaining to Ms. Kalen that her physical symptoms are not real.

11. Mr. Lin has a diagnosis of conversion disorder. He cannot see, even though no physical cause for blindness has been found. Which observation by the nurse would be most expected in a patient with a conversion disorder?

a. The client shows little concern about his blindness.
b. The client has a panic attack whenever his vision is discussed.

c. The client eagerly seeks psychiatric help for his problem.
d. The client is well liked by the nursing staff.

12. To reduce secondary gains for Mr. Lin, the nurse would:

a. Provide extra time to assist Mr. Lin with meals and other tasks that are difficult for the vision-impaired.
b. Make a daily assessment of Mr. Lin's vision and eye condition.
c. Focus attention on aspects of Mr. Lin's personality that are not part of his blindness.
d. Allow Mr. Lin to choose the activities in which he will participate.

ANSWERS

1. **Correct answer is a.** The initial nursing care for clients with severe and panic levels of anxiety must be directed at reducing the anxiety to a more manageable level. The nurse's presence and use of a calm, firm voice and simple instructions will help the client regain a sense of control.

b. Leaving a client with severe anxiety alone will intensify the anxiety.
c. A client with a high level of anxiety is unable to give information until the anxiety level has decreased.
d. The client's anxiety level is too high for her to think about coping mechanisms. The nurse's initial focus must be on reduction of the anxiety to a manageable level. When anxiety is high, the client cannot focus on complex concepts.

2. **Correct answer is b.** Clients taking antianxiety medications should also continue to learn better ways to cope with the anxiety.

a. Clients taking antianxiety medications should avoid use of alcohol, since it may potentiate CNS depression.
c. Caffeine will interfere with the action of alprazolam and may increase symptoms of anxiety; it should be avoided by clients

taking antianxiety medications and by clients with anxiety disorders.

d. Alprazolam may cause nausea if taken on an empty stomach; the client may find a light snack (such as crackers) helpful to relieve the upset stomach.

3. **Correct answer is c.** Panic is characterized by elevated heart rate, elevated blood pressure, tightness in the chest, hyperventilation, diaphoresis, urinary frequency, gastrointestinal disturbance, dizziness, and feelings of impending doom that appear suddenly and without a cause apparent to the client.

a. This statement is a description of an auditory hallucination, which would be an expected finding if the diagnosis were schizophrenia.
b. Insomnia without fatigue and an exaggerated feeling of importance are typical of the client with bipolar disorder, manic type.
d. Clients with somatization disorder describe a long history of illness and tend to express anxiety as a physical condition.

4. **Correct answer is a.** Ms. Ferrante's comment that she is less competent than her family is evidence of low self-esteem.

b. This comment supports a nursing diagnosis of social isolation (which may also be appropriate for Ms. Ferrante).
c. Use of a ritual to decrease anxiety supports a nursing diagnosis of ineffective individual coping. This nursing diagnosis is almost certain to be appropriate for Ms. Ferrante and other clients with obsessive-compulsive disorder.
d. Mr. Ferrante's attitude toward Ms. Ferrante may indicate a nursing diagnosis of altered family processes and could be a consideration in the client's care.

5. **Correct answer is c.** There are indications that hand washing is a ritual that decreases Ms. Ferrante's anxiety. If she is prevented from carrying out the ritual, she may experience panic. As her treatment progresses, the client's need for the ritual will

decrease, and she can assist in making plans to give it up.

a. Although it is important to help Ms. Ferrante find her positive attributes, allowing her to carry out rituals that decrease anxiety takes priority.
b. Attendance at group functions will help decrease Ms. Ferrante's social isolation, but early in her hospitalization the priority is to decrease her anxiety.
d. Joint counseling may be desirable, but it is not the first priority.

6. **Correct answer is c.** Desensitization involves using relaxation while increasing exposure to the anxiety-producing situation. The exposure can be through fantasy or through real experiences, but it should gradually increase in intensity.

a. Most individuals with phobias recognize that they are senseless and recognize when the phobia interferes with their life. Attempts by the nurse to "talk the client out of it" tend to lower the client's self-esteem further.
b. Social phobias are treatable. Mr. Harris should be encouraged to try treatment before he considers a career change.
d. Sudden exposure to a feared object or situation in an individual with phobias will likely precipitate a panic attack and will certainly destroy any trust that the client might have developed in the nurse.

7. **Correct answer is a.** The diagnosis of posttraumatic stress disorder requires that the client has experienced a traumatic event outside the normal range of human experience, followed by recurrent subjective reexperiencing of the event (which may take the form of nightmares or flashbacks).

b. A client with agoraphobia would be afraid to leave home.
c. A client with conversion disorder experiences loss or alteration of a physical function soon after experiencing stress.
d. Characteristics of the dissociative disorders include episodes of amnesia and identity problems.

8. **Correct answer is d.** Potential for violence must take priority so that Mr. Jankowicz does not hurt himself or anyone else.

a, b, and **c.** These may be appropriate nursing diagnoses for Mr. Jankowicz, but they are not the highest priority early in his treatment. His physical safety must come first.

9. **Correct answer is c.** Verbalizing memories of the trauma to listeners who are understanding can provide relief for the client with posttraumatic stress disorder. Often, peer support groups such as veterans' groups, rape crisis centers, or victim support groups can fill this need.

a. Antidepressant, antianxiety, or antipsychotic drugs may be prescribed to alleviate symptoms for the client with posttraumatic stress disorder, but they do not provide the lasting relief that ventilation to sympathetic listeners can offer.
b. Families are often both sympathetic to and frightened of the client with posttraumatic stress disorder. It is difficult for the family to bear the client's pain when he/she discusses the traumatic event; this is best left to a more neutral party.
d. Alcohol abuse is a common part of posttraumatic stress disorder and must be considered in planning treatment, but education alone will not relieve the symptoms of the disorder that lead the client to drink.

10. **Correct answer is c.** Before making the final diagnosis of somatization disorder and undertaking treatment, the health care team must ascertain that no physical illness exists. The nurse's role in this process includes recording pertinent observations and supporting the client through diagnostic procedures.

a. Clients with somatization disorder usually focus most of their conversation on their physical symptoms.
b. Once the diagnosis of somatization disorder has been finalized, this approach

might be a part of the treatment plan. It is inappropriate early in the hospitalization and will serve only to increase the client's symptoms and alienate her from the staff.
d. The nurse cannot know if the physical symptoms are real until diagnostic testing has been completed; even then it is essential to recognize that the symptoms are very real to the client, and explanations to the contrary may only alienate the client from the nurse.

11. **Correct answer is a.** Clients with conversion disorder often have la belle indifférence—a lack of concern about the physical symptom.

b. In conversion disorder, anxiety is channeled into the physical symptom, and the client appears unconcerned or less anxious than expected.
c. Clients with conversion disorder usually resist psychiatric help or psychologic explanations for their problems.
d. Nursing staff may respond to clients with conversion disorder with negative countertransference, expressed as anger, frustration, or insensitivity.

12. **Correct answer is c.** In conversion disorder, the primary gain is the removal of the psychologic conflict from awareness. The secondary gain is that the physical symptoms allow the client to avoid distressing activities while receiving support from others. Focusing attention away from the symptoms and toward healthy aspects of the personality can decrease the secondary gain.

a. Giving special attention because of the symptom increases the secondary gain from conversion disorder.
b. Once it has been established that the symptom has no physiologic basis, attention should be directed to healthier parts of the personality.
d. The client with conversion disorder should be expected to take part in the unit routine with few special privileges.

6

Schizophrenic Disorders

NURSING HIGHLIGHTS

1. Schizophrenia is not 1 but several related chronic disorders, all of which involve loss of contact with reality and irrational thinking.
2. The causes of schizophrenia are not well understood; however, the effectiveness of antipsychotic medications suggests a biochemical basis for the disease. An interrelationship between biologic and environmental factors is proposed.
3. Schizophrenia is treated primarily with antipsychotic drugs supplemented by psychotherapy and family therapy. Treatment is lifelong.
4. Key nursing care for clients with schizophrenia focuses on physical care and safety, monitoring for adverse effects of medications, helping the client reestablish contact with reality, and educating the family and client about the nature of the disease and the importance of taking medication as prescribed.
5. Caring for the client with schizophrenia is challenging and taxing; introspection and feedback from peers and supervisors are important to help the nurse develop optimal nursing skills for these clients.

GLOSSARY

agranulocytosis—acute condition in which decreased production of granulated white blood cells (leukocytes) leaves body defenseless against infection; usually caused by reaction to drugs that affect bone marrow

catatonia—condition characterized by disturbance in motor behavior, such as rigidity or extreme agitation

depersonalization—persistent feelings in which the self and the external world appear unreal

derealization—defense mechanism in which people, situations, and environment appear unreal; found in an extreme form in people with schizophrenia

extrapyramidal symptoms—reactions to antipsychotic medications that involve the extrapyramidal part of the central nervous system (the part that regulates muscle tone and motor functions)

galactorrhea—lactation not associated with childbirth or nursing

magical thinking—cognitive process based on the belief that the power of thought can influence events or outcomes

paranoia—condition in which an individual has persistent, systematized delusions (e.g., of persecution or grandeur), sometimes including the person's belief of superiority

reality checking—testing aspects of one's environment to verify the difference between external reality and internal world of fantasy

waxy flexibility—condition in which skeletal muscles become semirigid, allowing a person to remain in awkward, often bizarre, positions for long periods; often exhibited by people with schizophrenia during withdrawal

ENHANCED OUTLINE

I. General concepts

> See text pages
> _____

A. Symptoms of schizophrenia
  1. Primary symptoms or behaviors (Eugen Bleuler's 4 A's)
     a) Affective symptoms
        (1) Flatness or blunting of expression, including a decrease in intensity of emotional responses (e.g., monotone voice, few changes in facial expression)
        (2) Expression of inappropriate hostility
        (3) Inappropriate expression of feelings (e.g., laughing when discussing a traumatic event)
     b) Associative symptoms: disrupted thought processes and communication attempts
        (1) Blocking (also called thought deprivation): sudden, unexplained silences
        (2) Looseness of association: stringing together unrelated thoughts or words
        (3) Echolalia: automatically repeating exactly what another person has said
        (4) Word salad: using combinations of words that have no meaning
        (5) Circumstantiality: providing overly detailed responses
        (6) Clang associations: rhyming words without attention to meaning
     c) Autism: preoccupation with own needs and thoughts; possible creation of fantasy worlds; may be expressed through invented words (neologisms), head banging, hallucinations, or delusions

        d) Ambivalence: difficulty in making decisions or simultaneous experiencing of conflicting emotions

    2. Additional symptoms

        a) Behavioral symptoms

            (1) Withdrawal, perhaps leading to catatonic posturing (holding same, usually bizarre, position for long periods) or catatonic stupor (no response)

            (2) Negativism: doing the opposite of what is required or asked or not doing things that are necessary for life (e.g., eating, sleeping)

            (3) Mechanical motor activity (repeating the same action)

            (4) Echopraxia: mimicking the actions of others

            (5) Catatonic excitement: agitated movements not caused by external stimuli

        b) Cognitive and perceptual symptoms

            (1) Delusions: fixed false beliefs

                (a) Persecution (e.g., client's belief that someone is trying to kill him/her)

                (b) Grandeur (e.g., client's belief that God has singled him/her out)

                (c) Somatic (e.g., client's belief that he/she is suffering from a serious disease)

            (2) Hallucinations: sensory perceptions of objects, images, and sensations that occur in the absence of external stimuli

                (a) Auditory hallucination (e.g., hearing voices) is the most common type.

                (b) Other types are visual, olfactory, gustatory, tactile, and somatic.

                (c) According to anxiety model, hallucinations are attempts to reduce anxiety by shifting repressed thoughts to an "outside" source.

                (d) According to biologic models, hallucinations are caused by excess dopamine activity.

        c) Affective symptoms

            (1) Depression

            (2) Depersonalization

            (3) Derealization

B. Theories of causation

    1. Biologic theories

        a) Genetic studies show evidence of a hereditary component to schizophrenia.

b) Pathologic and clinical studies show some brain abnormalities (e.g., ventricular enlargement) among those with schizophrenia, but the studies indicate no consistent defects or specific understanding about why the abnormalities occur.

c) Research has shown a relationship between biochemical imbalances and schizophrenia.

    (1) Dopamine theory: Some cases of schizophrenia may be related to excessive amounts of the enzyme dopamine in the brain; currently, research into the effects of this neurotransmitter on the brain offers the most promising information about biochemical causes of schizophrenia.

    (2) Indolamine theory: This theory suggests that a defect in metabolism of the indolamine serotonin may be a cause of some cases of schizophrenia.

d) The information processing theory suggests that a primary deficit in the brain's information processing capabilities causes schizophrenic behavior.

2. Environmental theories

    a) Stressors appear to play a role in causing and/or triggering schizophrenia.

        (1) Psychologic stressors, either real or perceived (e.g., loss of control, isolation)

        (2) Sociocultural stressors (e.g., family or interpersonal problems)

    b) Developmental theory indicates that a person may develop schizophrenia if, as a child, he/she is not oriented to reality by the mother figure (i.e., if he/she is consistently unable to obtain realistic feedback [reality checking] regarding thoughts, feelings, and actions).

    c) Now discredited, the family theory held that parental behavior was a cause of schizophrenia; while it has been shown that parental influences do not cause the disease, they may play a role in the course of the disease (e.g., relapse).

C. Types (DSM-IV)

1. Schizophrenia: general features

    a) At least 2 of the following symptoms are present for a large part of 1 month:

        (1) Delusions

        (2) Hallucinations

        (3) Disorganized speech

        (4) Grossly disorganized or catatonic behavior

        (5) Negative symptoms (flattened affect, inability to speak, inability to make decisions)

    b) Only 1 symptom is needed if delusions are bizarre (could not happen in real life) or if auditory hallucinations are continuous or consist of at least 2 voices.

    c) Signs of disturbance last at least 6 months.

    d) Condition affects work or social functioning.

2. Subtypes of schizophrenia
   a) Paranoid type: preoccupation with 1 or more delusions or auditory hallucinations; no evidence of incoherence, loose associations, affective disturbances, catatonia, or gross disorganization
   b) Disorganized type: presence of incoherence, loose associations, gross disorganization of behavior, and flat or inappropriate affect; no evidence of catatonia
   c) Catatonic type: prevalence of at least 2 of the following sets of symptoms:
      (1) Catatonic stupor or rigidity (including waxy flexibility)
      (2) Catatonic excitement
      (3) Mutism or negativism
      (4) Bizarre voluntary movements (e.g., catatonic posturing, grimacing)
      (5) Echolalia or echopraxia
   d) Undifferentiated type: 2 or more of the general features of schizophrenia: delusions, hallucinations, disorganized speech, grossly disorganized or catatonic behavior, or a negative symptom (flattened affect, inability to speak, or inability to decide)
   e) Residual type
      (1) Client does not experience active-phase symptoms (e.g., delusions, hallucinations, incoherence, gross disorganization) or other general symptoms of schizophrenia.
      (2) Client exhibits negative symptoms or active-phase symptoms in reduced form (e.g., marked social isolation or withdrawal, markedly impaired role function, markedly peculiar behavior, marked impairment in personal hygiene or grooming, blunted or inappropriate affect, odd beliefs or magical thinking, unusual perceptual experiences, or apathy). Features do not fully interfere with client's ability to function.

D. Related psychotic disorders (DSM-IV): those having some clinical symptoms of schizophrenia
   1. Schizophreniform disorder (with or without good prognostic features): schizophrenialike symptoms lasting at least 1 month but less than 6 months; return to normal functioning possible
   2. Schizoaffective disorder: schizophrenialike symptoms accompanied at some point by a major depressive episode or manic episode
   3. Delusional disorder: delusional thinking that is not bizarre and that lasts at least 1 month
   4. Brief psychotic disorder: delusions, hallucinations, disorganized speech, and grossly disorganized or catatonic speech lasting at least 1 day but not more than 1 month; may occur shortly after a stressful event or series of events (called brief reactive) or after no marked stressful event

5. Shared psychotic disorder (called induced psychotic disorder in DSM-III-R): delusional symptoms occurring because of a close relationship with another person who has delusions; also referred to as folie à deux
6. Psychotic disorder due to general medical condition
7. Substance-induced psychotic disorder
8. Psychotic disorder not otherwise specified

II. Treatments

A. Antipsychotic medications
  1. Traditional neuroleptics
    a) Classes
      (1) Phenothiazines (e.g., chlorpromazine [Thorazine])
      (2) Thioxanthenes (e.g., thiothixene [Navane])
      (3) Butyrophenones (e.g., haloperidol [Haldol])
      (4) Dibenzoxazepines (e.g., loxapine hydrochloride [Loxitane])
      (5) Dihydroindolones (e.g., molindone hydrochloride [Moban])
    b) Benefits
      (1) Some degree of help for about 90% of clients with schizophrenia; usually begin working within 3–6 weeks
      (2) Reduction in hostile, disruptive, and assaultive behaviors
      (3) Increase in activity, speech, and sociability in withdrawn clients
      (4) Improvement in self-care and insomnia
      (5) Improvement in positive symptoms of schizophrenia
        (a) Lessening of occurrence of such thought processes as loose associations, suspiciousness, paranoia, and negativism
        (b) Control of hallucinations and delusions, either by eliminating them or by reducing fear and anxiety that they cause
      (6) Unlikely to cause lethal overdose
    c) Risks and cautions
      (1) Effects on autonomic nervous system (greater incidence with low-potency drugs such as chlorpromazine than with high-potency drugs such as haloperidol): postural, or orthostatic, hypotension (systolic pressure of 80); urinary retention; constipation; blurred vision; dry mouth; skin allergies; sensitivity to sun; weight gain; male impotence; female menstrual irregularities; galactorrhea
      (2) Extrapyramidal symptoms (EPS) (those affecting extrapyramidal part of central nervous system [CNS]): greater incidence of EPS with high-potency drugs such as haloperidol than with low-potency drugs such as chlorpromazine
        (a) Akathisia (pacing, agitation, and fidgeting): may happen during first few days of therapy or weeks or months after treatment has begun; reversible with change of antipsychotic drug or with administration of an anticholinergic or muscle relaxant; may be mistaken for anxiety or agitation

See text pages
_____

        (b) Pseudoparkinsonism (stiffening of muscles in face, body, and limbs; tremors; drooling; shuffling walk): reversible with change to lower dosage or to another drug or with administration of an anticholinergic

        (c) Acute dystonia (spasms of head, neck, back, and limbs and abnormal eye movements): temporary side effect, usually during first few days of therapy; frightening and painful for client; alleviated by injection of an anticholinergic

        (d) Tardive dyskinesia (TD): severe and possibly irreversible; usually occurs with long-term use of high doses of antipsychotic drugs, often when dose is discontinued or reduced; elderly women at particular risk; no reliable treatment; prevention is key, including periodic screening for TD with use of the Abnormal Involuntary Movement Scale (AIMS) (see Nurse Alert, "Symptoms of Tardive Dyskinesia")

   (3) Other effects on CNS: increased likelihood of seizure activity or sedation

   (4) Neuroleptic malignant syndrome (NMS)

        (a) Develops quickly (1–3 days); sometimes fatal; relatively rare

        (b) May affect clients who are receiving long-term maintenance doses or who have just started drug program; may be related to high-potency drugs

        (c) May affect clients who are dehydrated

! NURSE *ALERT* !

Symptoms of Tardive Dyskinesia

Watch for the following signs and symptoms of tardive dyskinesia; call them to the attention of the physician, who may order changes in the antipsychotic medication or dosage or discontinuation of treatment:

- Involuntary muscle spasms of fingers, toes, neck, trunk, or pelvis
- Protruding tongue, puffed cheeks, or puckered lips
- Eye twitching
- Drooling
- Difficulty swallowing and neck stiffness
- Slow, repetitive movements of arms and legs
- Twitching
- Bizarre grimacing

NOTE: Document signs and symptoms for comparison during future hospitalizations, because tardive dyskinesia can develop insidiously.

           (d) Symptoms: may include very high fever (up to 107°F), diaphoresis, severe rigidity, elevated white blood cell (WBC) count, increase in liver enzymes, unstable blood pressure, altered consciousness, renal shutdown

           (e) Requires discontinuance of drug and treatment of symptoms (e.g., dialysis for renal failure, ice packs to reduce fever, techniques to improve hydration)

      (5) Agranulocytosis

           (a) Potentially fatal; may be reversible if detected early (within 1–2 weeks of onset)

           (b) Particularly at risk: geriatric females

           (c) Symptoms: infection, high fever, chills, prostration, ulceration of mucous membranes, sore throat, malaise, WBC count $<500/mm^3$

           (d) Requires discontinuance of drug, which cannot be resumed

  2. Clozapine (Clozaril): atypical antipsychotic agent

    a) Clozapine offers benefits to clients who do not respond to traditional neuroleptic antipsychotics; it offers relief from both positive symptoms (hallucinations, delusions, and disordered thought processes) and negative symptoms (apathy, flattened affect, and poverty of thought) of schizophrenia.

    b) Clozapine may cause a number of side effects; particularly serious is agranulocytosis (see section II,A,1,c,5 of this chapter and Nurse Alert, "Side Effects of Clozapine [Clozaril]").

B. Individual and group psychotherapy

C. Family therapy

! NURSE *ALERT* !

Side Effects of Clozapine (Clozaril)

Serious side effects of clozapine use are:

- Agranulocytosis
- Seizure potential
- Sedation
- Tachycardia
- Orthostatic hypotension

Possible signs of infection, such as lethargy, fever, sore throat, malaise, and ulceration of mucous membranes, should be reported to the client's physician immediately.

NOTE: Clozapine is dispensed through prescriptions that are limited to a 1-week supply. Clients receiving clozapine are required to have weekly blood tests to monitor white blood cell (WBC) counts so that agranulocytosis can be identified in its early stages. Only with proof of a satisfactory blood test will the next week's supply be dispensed. WBC counts $<2000/mm^3$ or granulocyte counts $<1000/mm^3$ call for discontinuance of the drug; these clients must not resume clozapine therapy.

DEPARTMENT OF HEALTH AND HUMAN SERVICES
PUBLIC HEALTH SERVICE
Alcohol, Drug Abuse, and Mental Health Administration
NIMH Treatment Strategies in Schizophrenia Study

**ABNORMAL INVOLUNTARY
MOVEMENT SCALE
(AIMS)**

PATIENT NUMBER | DATA GROUP | EVALUATION DATE

— — — — aims M M - D D - Y Y

PATIENT NAME

RATER NAME

RATER NUMBER

— — —

EVALUATION TYPE *(Circle)*

1 Baseline	4 Start double-blind	7 Start open meds	10 Early termination
2 2-week minor	5 Major evaluation	8 During open meds	11 Study completion
3	6 Other	9 Stop open meds	

INSTRUCTIONS: Complete Examination Procedure (reverse side) before making ratings.
MOVEMENT RATINGS: Rate highest severity observed.

Code: 1 = None
2 = Minimal, may be extreme normal
3 = Mild
4 = Moderate
5 = Severe

			(Circle One)				
FACIAL AND ORAL MOVEMENTS:	1.	**Muscles of Facial Expression** e.g., movements of forehead, eyebrows, periorbital area, cheeks; include frowning, blinking, smiling, grimacing	1	2	3	4	5
	2.	**Lips and Perioral Area** e.g., puckering, pouting, smacking	1	2	3	4	5
	3.	**Jaw** e.g., biting, clenching, chewing, mouth opening, lateral movement	1	2	3	4	5
	4.	**Tongue** Rate only increase in movement both in and out of mouth, NOT inability to sustain movement	1	2	3	4	5
EXTREMITY MOVEMENTS:	5.	**Upper** *(arms, wrists, hands, fingers)* Include choreic movements, (i.e., rapid, objectively purposeless, irregular, spontaneous), athetoid movements (i.e., slow, irregular, complex, serpentine). Do NOT include tremor (i.e., repetitive, regular, rhythmic)	1	2	3	4	5
	6.	**Lower** *(legs, knees, ankles, toes)* e.g., lateral knee movement, foot tapping, heel dropping, foot squirming, inversion and eversion of foot	1	2	3	4	5
TRUNK MOVEMENTS:	7.	**Neck, shoulders, hips** e.g., rocking, twisting, squirming, pelvic gyrations	1	2	3	4	5
GLOBAL JUDGMENTS:	8.	Severity of abnormal movements	None, normal 1 Minimal 2 Mild 3 Moderate 4 Severe 5				
	9.	Incapacitation due to abnormal movements	None, normal 1 Minimal 2 Mild 3 Moderate 4 Severe 5				
	10.	Patient's awareness of abnormal movements Rate only patient's report	No awareness 1 Aware, no distress 2 Aware, mild distress 3 Aware, moderate distress 4 Aware, severe distress 5				
DENTAL STATUS:	11.	Current problems with teeth and/or dentures	No 1 Yes 2				
	12.	Does patient usually wear dentures?	No 1 Yes 2				

ADM 117
Rev. 11-85

Figure 6–1
AIMS Test for Tardive Dyskinesia

Either before or after completing the Examination Procedure observe the patient unobtrusively, at rest (e.g., in waiting room).

The chair to be used in this examination should be a hard, firm one without arms.

1. Ask patient to remove shoes and socks.

2. Ask patient whether there is anything in his/her mouth (i.e., gum, candy, etc.) and if there is, to remove it.

3. Ask patient about the current condition of his/her teeth. Ask patient if he/she wears dentures. Do teeth or dentures bother patient now?

4. Ask patient whether he/she notices any movements in mouth, face, hands, or feet. If yes, ask to describe and to what extent they currently bother patient or interfere with his/her activities.

5. Have patient sit in chair with hands on knees, legs slightly apart, and feet flat on floor. (Look at entire body for movements while in this position.)

6. Ask patient to sit with hands hanging unsupported. If male, between legs, if female and wearing a dress, hanging over knees. (Observe hands and other body areas.)

7. Ask patient to open mouth. (Observe tongue at rest within mouth.) Do this twice.

8. Ask patient to protrude tongue. (Observe abnormalities of tongue movement.) Do this twice.

9. Ask patient to tap thumb, with each finger, as rapidly as possible for 10-15 seconds; separately with right hand, then with left hand. (Observe facial and leg movements.)

10. Flex and extend patient's left and right arms (one at a time). (Note any rigidity.)

11. Ask patient to stand up. (Observe in profile. Observe all body areas again, hips included.)

12. Ask patient to extend both arms outstretched in front with palms down. (Observe trunk, legs, and mouth.)

13. Have patient walk a few paces, turn, and walk back to chair. (Observe hands and gait.) Do this twice.

ADM-9 117 (Back)
12-84

PAGE 2

Figure 6–1
AIMS Test for Tardive Dyskinesia (continued)

See text pages

_____

III. Essential nursing care

A. Nursing assessment
1. Record observations of client's behavior and affect.
2. Assess symptoms: physical, behavioral, affective, and cognitive.
3. Collect data to differentiate between schizophrenia and physical and psychologic disorders that produce symptoms resembling schizophrenia.
4. Assess potential for client to harm self or others.

B. Nursing diagnoses
1. Main NANDA nursing diagnoses
   a) Ineffective individual coping
   b) Self-esteem disturbance
   c) Altered thought processes
   d) Social isolation
2. Additional NANDA nursing diagnoses
   a) Impaired adjustment
   b) Anxiety
   c) Impaired verbal communication
   d) Altered sensory perceptions
   e) Altered role performance
   f) Decisional conflict
   g) Activity intolerance
   h) Potential for violence, self-directed or directed at others
   i) Ineffective family coping
   j) Altered family processes
   k) Noncompliance with medications
   l) Self-care deficits
   m) Body image disturbance
   n) Altered nutrition, less than body requirements
3. Selected complete nursing diagnoses
   a) Ineffective individual coping related to distrust of others evidenced by unwillingness to provide information for client history
   b) Altered thought processes related to hallucinations evidenced by report that voices are telling client what to do

C. Planning (goal setting)
1. General goals
   a) Promote a safe environment.
   b) Promote client's growth toward achieving maximum functional status.
   c) Promote and support rational behavior and thought.
   d) Help client establish meaningful communication patterns.

e) Promote and support client's ability to engage in meaningful relationships with others.

f) Educate client (to extent possible) and family about the client's condition and treatment; emphasize need for compliance with drug regimens and other aspects of treatment plan.

g) Promote and support client's integration into his/her family and community.

2. Examples of specific goals

a) Client will maintain adequate nutrition and hydration.

b) Client will engage in interactions with the nursing staff without echolalia or looseness of association.

c) Client will identify feelings of anger and express them appropriately when they occur during interactions with the nursing staff.

d) Client will meet with nurse and another client to engage in card games or other social or interactive activities.

e) Client will take medications as ordered when in an outpatient setting.

D. Nursing implementation (intervention)

1. Maintain client's biologic integrity: Clients with schizophrenia are often unable to meet their basic physical needs for food and fluid intake.

a) Monitor and record food and fluid intake.

b) Record output to identify urinary and fecal retention.

c) Provide intravenous or tube feeding if ordered and required.

d) If invasive measures are required, explain to client that they are necessary for his/her health and are not punishments.

e) If client refuses to move voluntarily, turn client, and provide skin care to prevent skin breakdown and pressure ulcers.

f) When administering oral medication, be sure that the client has swallowed it; paranoid or suspicious clients may attempt to avoid taking prescribed medication.

2. Protect client from harming self or others.

a) Monitor behavior.

b) Alert physician to behavior or statements suggesting increased risk of harm and possible need for restraint, seclusion, or increased observation.

c) Remove sharp objects and other potentially dangerous items if client is at risk for aggressive or assaultive behavior.

d) Use physical restraints only upon a physician's orders.

e) Assess and record physical and psychologic effects of restraint and/or seclusion.

3. Administer medication as ordered, and monitor for effectiveness and side effects.

a) Establish a baseline blood pressure before beginning medications.

b) Check blood pressure before giving antipsychotic drug to monitor for the side effect of postural hypotension.

c) Observe and record objective and subjective changes in the client.

      d) Watch for side effects, especially signs of akathisia, tardive dyskinesia, neuroleptic malignant syndrome, and agranulocytosis.

      e) Reassure client that temporary side effects will pass; if possible, stay with client when upsetting side effects, such as those of acute dystonia, occur; and when client is an outpatient, encourage compliance until frightening side effects can be overcome.

4. Facilitate communication. (See Chapter 2, section VI,B,5, for facilitative communication strategies.)

      a) Communicate with client even if he/she does not respond; keep in mind that clients with schizophrenia are often aware of their surroundings even when they are not responsive.

      b) Remain nonjudgmental in the face of hostility or rejection.

      c) Give feedback to client; let client know when you do not understand what he/she is saying.

      d) Engage in goal-directed communication; use topics and conversational styles (e.g., open-ended statements, pauses) that will promote the client's participation.

      e) Use direct questioning with caution, since it may increase the client's anxiety.

      f) Provide client with the opportunity to make appropriate choices (e.g., choosing his/her clothes for the day).

      g) Use clear, concise language and a matter-of-fact approach; avoid "talking down" to the client.

      h) Be aware of and respond to the client's nonverbal communication (e.g., body posture, gestures, eye contact).

      i) Use nonverbal communication to make contact with client (e.g., eye contact, body posture).

      j) Use touch cautiously; it may increase the client's anxiety.

      k) Keep nurse-client interactions brief, especially in the beginning.

5. Promote rational thought and expression.

      a) Implement interventions for delusional thinking.

         (1) Do not attack or belittle client's delusions; doing so may increase anxiety levels.

         (2) Express doubts about the delusion, and shift the focus to the client's feelings (e.g., "Often when people are afraid or in an unfamiliar place, they have the feeling that someone is out to get them").

      b) Implement interventions for hallucinations.

         (1) Monitor client for precipitating stressors.

         (2) Assess client needs that are related to the underlying anxiety.

         (3) Using client's verbal and nonverbal cues, recognize client's feelings that are associated with the hallucinations, and acknowledge these feelings to the client.

       (4) Cast doubt on the reality of hallucinations by telling client that you do not hear or see them (e.g., "I know these voices frighten you; I want you to know that I don't hear them").

       (5) Encourage client to talk about reality-based issues, such as his/her fears and anxieties or everyday topics such as the weather.

       (6) As trust grows between client and nurse, encourage client to dismiss the voices by telling them to go away or be quiet.

6. Provide structure for the client.
   a) Give clear direction.
   b) Provide schedule of activities, and stick to it.
   c) Provide positive reinforcement.

7. Promote decision making.
   a) Limit choices to avoid overwhelming the client.
   b) Give client responsibility for simple self-care tasks to the extent possible; provide instruction and guidance as necessary.
   c) Introduce more complex tasks as simple ones are mastered.
   d) Encourage client to develop new skills.
   e) Help client and family understand and practice the steps in the decision-making process.
      (1) Identify the problem.
      (2) List alternatives.
      (3) Evaluate alternatives.
      (4) Test the chosen alternative.

8. Facilitate social participation.
   a) Gradually expand the client's social network.
      (1) Bring third parties into discussions and activities.
      (2) Introduce client to other clients.
   b) If present, help the client overcome resistance to involvement with the staff.

9. Provide client education in preparation for outpatient status.
   a) Help client identify concerns related to expression of feelings.
   b) Help client explore the meaning of experiencing pleasure.
   c) Help client explore concepts related to anxiety.
   d) Help client learn stress reduction techniques.
   e) Provide client with accurate information about the schizophrenia disease process.
   f) Provide client with information about symptoms and medications.
   g) Provide referrals to community providers, organizations, and support groups.

10. Provide family with information (see Client Teaching Checklist, "Family of Individual with Schizophrenia").

11. As the nurse-client relationship terminates or changes, help client explore feelings of loss and change.

E. Nursing evaluation
   1. Obtain objective and subjective validation of the effectiveness of the nurse-client relationship.
      a) A supervisor or clinical nurse specialist can help the nurse gain insights into the therapeutic relationship with the client.

b) Introspection and feedback from other team members and family also provide information about the success of the therapeutic relationship.

2. Evaluate the client's behavioral changes continuously, using feedback from the client, health care team, and family.

3. Review goals, and assess progress.
   a) Client was included in treatment decisions.
   b) Client's biologic needs are met.
   c) Client's communication skills improve.
   d) Client exhibits rational thought and expression.
   e) Client's decision-making skills improve and are adequate.
   f) Client's social interaction and support systems improve.
   g) Client and family understand the disease process and when they should seek additional help.
   h) Referrals have been made to appropriate sources of help and support within the community.
   i) Nurse-client relationship is terminated in a way that promotes positive growth for the client.

4. Revise goals and care plan as necessary.

✔ CLIENT TEACHING CHECKLIST ✔

Family of Individual with Schizophrenia

A key element in the nursing plan is to provide accurate and objective information to the family of the person who has schizophrenia.

✔ Encourage the family to learn as much as possible about the disease and about the treatment program, including the medications.

✔ Help family members explore their feelings about guilt and responsibility. These feelings may prompt denial or other behaviors that interfere with the family's ability to provide support and care for the client. To assess understanding, ask family members why they think the client developed schizophrenia. Correct any misperceptions that parenting methods have caused the disease. Help family members understand that they will be better able to help the client if they accept the fact that they are not to blame for the client's illness.

✔ Suggest that the family join a family support group or self-help group to avoid feelings of isolation.

✔ Discourage family members from sacrificing their own interests and pursuits as they care for the ill family member.

✔ Encourage family to practice stress reduction techniques and adaptive coping mechanisms.

✔ Help family members understand the level of functioning of the ill family member (especially one who is an outpatient) to avoid frustration.

1. Autistic thinking by the client with a diagnosis of schizophrenia is frequently exhibited through which of the following behaviors?

   a. Neologisms
   b. Negativism
   c. Automatic obedience
   d. Stupor

2. Interventions with clients who have delusions are most likely to be effective when the nurse:

   a. Shows disapproval of the delusional thoughts.
   b. Provides education about psychotic disorders.
   c. Can prove that the delusion is false.
   d. Focuses on reality-based topics.

3. Which of the following should be the initial nursing goal for a client who has schizophrenia?

   a. To develop a trusting relationship
   b. To improve self-care
   c. To limit bizarre behavior
   d. To encourage expression of feelings

4. Raymond, a client who has been diagnosed with paranoid schizophrenia, is admitted to the inpatient psychiatric unit. He is suspicious and withdrawn and is pacing up and down the hall. For which potential problem should the nurse assess first?

   a. Confusion
   b. Aggressive behavior
   c. Apathy
   d. Nutritional deficits

5. Which nursing intervention is most likely to foster a therapeutic relationship with Raymond?

   a. Leaving Raymond alone so that he does not feel pressured to interact with the nurse

   b. Confronting Raymond about his suspicious behavior
   c. Scheduling Raymond for a therapy group so that he can focus on external factors
   d. Meeting with Raymond briefly every day to discuss his concerns

6. At times, Raymond laughs uncontrollably though the nurse hasn't said anything funny. Which statement by the nurse is most appropriate in these situations?

   a. "You're laughing, Raymond. Tell me what's happening."
   b. "Raymond, I didn't say anything to make you laugh."
   c. "Were you thinking of a joke just now, Raymond?"
   d. "Why are you laughing, Raymond? What's so funny?"

7. Which client teaching statement made by the nurse provides essential information to a client taking clozapine (Clozaril)?

   a. Report fever or infection immediately.
   b. Monitor your salt intake.
   c. Monitor fluid intake closely to stabilize blood levels.
   d. Always take your medication with food.

8. Jill, a client with a diagnosis of chronic schizophrenia, does not shower regularly and wears the same clothing day after day. Which intervention by the nurse is most likely to improve Jill's hygiene?

   a. "Jill, would you like a shower today? You will feel so much better if you do."
   b. "Jill, it's time to shower now. Let's select some clean clothes first."
   c. "Jill, you must shower each morning. It is the policy on this unit."
   d. "Jill, can you tell me why you do not like to shower?"

9. During the first week of treatment, Jill's medication is increased, lessening her preoccupation with auditory hallucinations. Which plan is most appropriate as her mental status improves?

   a. Participate in community meeting daily
   b. Attend insight therapy group weekly
   c. Understand her relationship with her mother
   d. Maintain a daily journal of her feelings

10. When assessing for pseudoparkinsonism, a side effect of antipsychotic medication, the nurse observes for:

    a. Shuffling gait.
    b. High fever.
    c. Sudden, jerking movements.
    d. Labile affect.

11. Pseudoparkinsonism is usually managed by:

    a. Reassurance and supportive counseling.
    b. Discontinuation of antipsychotic medication.
    c. Addition of an anticholinergic medication.
    d. Relaxation techniques.

12. The nurse includes family education in the discharge teaching plan for a client who has schizophrenia because:

    a. Family members are expected to provide primary care for the client.
    b. The cause of schizophrenia has been traced to parental dysfunction.
    c. Relapse rates for clients who have schizophrenia are affected by family communication patterns.
    d. Outpatient services are not effective for clients who have schizophrenia, and symptoms may reappear.

ANSWERS

1. **Correct answer is a.** Neologisms are words constructed by the client that have special significance and meaning understood only by the client.

   b. Negativism is a disturbance in behavior in which the client either refuses to cooperate or does the opposite of the expected behavior.
   c. Automatic obedience is a disturbance in behavior in which a catatonic client follows simple commands in a robotlike fashion.
   d. Stupor is a disturbance in behavior in which the client is motionless and appears to be in a coma.

2. **Correct answer is d.** Since delusions defend against anxiety, the client will maintain the delusional thoughts until the anxiety is decreased through treatment. Focusing on reality-based topics helps minimize the client's internal preoccupation and encourage interaction with the environment.

   a. Showing disapproval is judgmental and nontherapeutic for a client in an anxiety state. It will increase client's fear and distrust of reality.
   b. It is unlikely that a client experiencing delusions would be able to learn, due to the preoccupation with internal thoughts and to the level of anxiety.
   c. By definition, delusions are false, fixed beliefs that the client retains despite evidence to the contrary. The client's reality testing is impaired due to the illness. It is nontherapeutic to pressure the client to give up this defense prematurely.

3. **Correct answer is a.** Difficulty with trusting is a primary feature of schizophrenia. Trust must be established before any therapeutic interventions can occur.

   b. Clients with a diagnosis of schizophrenia frequently ignore their self-care. Self-care is an appropriate goal after a trusting relationship has been established.
   c. Clients who have schizophrenia frequently demonstrate bizarre behavior until their medication takes effect. Since it can take 3–5 weeks for an antipsychotic medication to become effective, this goal would be appropriate later in the client's care.

d. Clients with a diagnosis of schizophrenia are usually unable to express or recognize their feelings until much later in treatment.

4. **Correct answer is b.** A client who has paranoia may misinterpret reality and feel threatened by normal interactions with the environment. This can result in aggressive behavior.

   a. The client who has paranoia may experience some confusion, but it is not the first concern of the nurse.

   c. Apathy is a common symptom of all types of schizophrenia and is addressed throughout treatment.

   d. Clients with a diagnosis of schizophrenia may or may not have nutritional deficits. The latter can be assessed for after the assessment for aggressive behavior has been made.

5. **Correct answer is d.** Regular meetings with the client provide structure. Allowing the client to set the agenda to include his concerns is supportive and develops trust.

   a. Avoiding contact with the client will encourage isolation and autistic thinking. The nurse provides opportunities for interaction with the environment.

   b. Confrontation will result in the client's becoming fearful and defensive. It is nontherapeutic early in the relationship.

   c. The client who has paranoia is unlikely to participate in a group setting until his anxiety decreases. Individual meetings that develop trust precede the group work.

6. **Correct answer is a.** Open-ended statements allow the client to describe what he is experiencing. This statement describes reality as observed by the nurse without making any assumptions about what the client is thinking.

   b. With this statement, the nurse is assuming that the client's response relates to their interaction. When clients experience autistic thinking, as those with schizophrenia do, their responses may be unrelated to the external stimulus.

c. A closed-ended question will not allow client to express what he is thinking.

d. Explanations made by a client who has schizophrenia about his autistic thoughts are frequently nonproductive and usually cannot be understood.

7. **Correct answer is a.** Clients taking clozapine (Clozaril) are at high risk for agranulocytosis. This side effect may cause infection and high fever. It can be fatal.

   b. Clozaril is not affected by salt intake.

   c. Clozaril is not affected by fluid intake.

   d. Food does not affect the bioavailability of clozapine.

8. **Correct answer is b.** This statement offers direct support for the client. The nurse is becoming involved in the client's care.

   a. Clients with a diagnosis of schizophrenia have a difficult time making decisions. Therefore, Jill may be unable to answer the nurse's question.

   c. Negative symptoms of schizophrenia impair a client's ability to act assertively. It is unlikely that unit policy will motivate Jill to take a shower without direct intervention by the nurse.

   d. It is difficult for clients who have schizophrenia to explain their behavior because they usually lack insight and abstract thinking.

9. **Correct answer is a.** Community meeting is a structured part of the treatment for clients whose acute schizophrenic symptoms have abated somewhat. Community meetings, which address community living issues, are usually nonthreatening and concrete. Participation helps the client focus on external surroundings.

   b. Insight therapy is usually not the treatment of choice for clients who have schizophrenia.

   c. Although relationship issues are important in the client's care, treatment during the first week focuses mainly on stabilizing the psychosis.

d. Clients who have schizophrenia are usually internally focused and need redirection to external issues. Later in treatment, it may be appropriate for Jill to keep a journal of her feelings.

10. **Correct answer is a.** Shuffling gait is a symptom of pseudoparkinsonism. Pseudoparkinsonism is identical in appearance to parkinsonism, but it is induced by antipsychotic medications.

    b. High fever is not a sign of pseudoparkinsonism.
    c. With pseudoparkinsonism, the client generally experiences muscle rigidity and has slow voluntary movements, not sudden, jerking movements.
    d. With pseudoparkinsonism, the client displays a masklike face and an apathetic appearance.

11. **Correct answer is c.** Anticholinergic medications such as benztropine mesylate (Cogentin) or diphenhydramine hydrochloride (Benadryl) are most commonly used to manage pseudoparkinsonism.

    a. Although support and reassurance may be helpful to a client with pseudoparkinsonism, the problem requires medical intervention.

    b. Since pseudoparkinsonism is not life-threatening, medication is normally continued, with the addition of an anticholinergic agent. If the symptoms are too distressing for the client, a different antipsychotic medication might be tried.
    d. Relaxation techniques are not effective in managing pseudoparkinsonism.

12. **Correct answer is c.** Research studies have identified that when communication patterns in the families of clients who have schizophrenia include a great degree of hostility and negativism, the client relapses more frequently. Family education about this fact may help address the problem and avoid relapse.

    a. Family members are encouraged to support the client's participation in outpatient services and to utilize community providers and organizations, but they are not expected to provide primary care.
    b. The theory of causation that points to parental behaviors as being the cause of schizophrenia has never been proven.
    d. Most clients who have schizophrenia are managed in outpatient settings. Although symptoms may reappear, early recognition may avoid hospitalization.

7

Mood Disorders

NURSING HIGHLIGHTS

1. Mood disorders involve prolonged and severe disturbances of the emotions, which disrupt normal social and psychologic functioning; mood disorders do not, however, impair rational thought or perception.
2. Clinical mood disorders generally involve episodes of depression, mania, and/or incomplete or delayed grieving.
3. While psychotherapeutic interventions play a role in the treatment of depression and mania, the primary means of treatment is with drug therapy (antidepressants and lithium).
4. Nurse encounters and can facilitate the normal grieving process in a variety of settings with both clients and families.
5. Nursing care plays a key role in the treatment of mood disorders by helping to create a therapeutic environment and by assisting the client in reestablishing social and life skills.

GLOSSARY

depression—an emotional state of excessive and/or persistent sadness; may range from mild dejection to extreme despair; one of the most common mental health problems

grief—state of sadness in response to a real or perceived loss such as separation from or death of a loved person or the loss of a job, a possession, self-
confidence, or a belief; may also be a response to loss of bodily function or
body part

lithium—medication based on a naturally occurring salt that acts as a mood
stabilizer for clients with mania by altering neurotransmitter actions

mania—pathologic state in which mood is abnormally elevated, expansive, ex-
cited, or irritable; impairs concentration

monoamine oxidase inhibitors (MAOIs)—antidepressant medications
that inhibit the metabolism of the neurotransmitters serotonin and norepinephrine at the presynaptic neuron in the central nervous system; also inhibit metabolism of tyramine

mood—prolonged emotional state that influences one's entire personality and
life functioning; also called affect, emotion, and feeling state

tricyclic antidepressants—medications that regulate the supply of the neurotransmitters serotonin and norepinephrine to the central nervous system

ENHANCED OUTLINE

See text pages
_____

I. General concepts

A. Grief reactions
   1. Normal grief reaction: a universal and healthy response to loss that
      progresses through specific stages and ends with acceptance of the loss
      (stages not always in order)
      a) Acute stage (4–8 weeks)
         (1) Shock, disbelief, and denial: normally lasts a few hours to a
             few days
         (2) Realization of the reality and permanence of the loss
             (a) Anger
             (b) Guilt
             (c) Physical symptoms of discomfort (e.g., pain in chest,
                 digestive disruptions)
             (d) Crying
         (3) Farewell ritual (e.g., funeral service)
      b) Long-term stage (symptoms possibly episodic for 1–2 years):
         Episodes may occur on anniversary dates or birthdays or when
         grieving person is in a new situation.
         (1) Physical illness
         (2) Guilt
         (3) Anger
         (4) Preoccupation with person who died or object of loss
         (5) Behavioral changes (e.g., disorganization, restlessness, despair)

c) Reorganization stage: behavioral adjustment
   (1) Formation of new relationships
   (2) Reestablishment of relationship with environment
2. Unresolved grief reactions: maladaptive responses to loss
  a) Delayed grief reaction: suppression or incompletion of the normal healthy grieving process
  b) Prolonged grief reaction: excessive preoccupation with the object of loss beyond the normal grieving period
  c) May lead to physical illness and mood disturbances, especially depression

B. General symptoms
  1. Symptoms of depression
   a) Fatigue or lethargy
   b) Suicidal thoughts
   c) Loss of interest and enjoyment
   d) Feeling of inadequacy and low self-esteem
   e) Helplessness
   f) Loss of motivation
   g) Indecisiveness
   h) Pessimism
   i) Sleeping or eating disorder
   j) Psychomotor retardation
  2. Symptoms of mania
   a) Egotism
   b) Aggressiveness
   c) Elation or euphoria
   d) Hyperactivity (social, sexual, verbal)
   e) Irritability
   f) Excessiveness of action or thought
   g) Insomnia
   h) Inadequate nutrition

C. Types of depressive disorders (DSM-IV)
  1. Major depressive episode
   a) At least 5 (including either depressed mood or loss of interest or pleasure) of the following symptoms occurring daily or almost daily during a 2-week period:
    (1) Depressed mood most of the day (may be irritable mood in children or adolescents)
    (2) Marked lessening of interest or pleasure in all or almost all activities
    (3) Significant loss or gain of weight or increase or decrease in appetite
    (4) Insomnia or excessive sleeping
    (5) Psychomotor agitation or slowness
    (6) Fatigue or lack of energy
    (7) Feelings of worthlessness or excessive guilt
    (8) Diminished ability to think or concentrate
    (9) Thoughts of death or suicide or a plan for suicide

        b) Includes symptoms causing clinically significant distress or social or job impairment

        c) May be a single episode or may be recurrent

        d) May range from mild to severe, with or without psychotic features

    2. Dysthymic disorder

        a) Depressed mood for most of the day and for more days than not for 2 years in adults and for 1 year in children and adolescents

        b) At least 3 of the following symptoms, along with depression:

           (1) Low self-esteem, low self-confidence, or feelings of inadequacy

           (2) Feelings of pessimism, despair, or hopelessness

           (3) Loss of interest or pleasure

           (4) Withdrawal

           (5) Chronic fatigue

           (6) Feelings of guilt or brooding about the past

           (7) Subjective irritability or excessive anger

           (8) Lessening of activity or productivity

           (9) Poor concentration or memory and ineffectiveness

        c) May be expressed as irritability in children and adolescents

        d) Onset

           (1) Early: before age 21

           (2) Late: age 21 or older

    3. Depressive disorder not otherwise specified: disorder (e.g., premenstrual dysphoric disorder) with depressive features that does not meet criteria for specific disorder

  D. Types of bipolar disorders (DSM-IV)

    1. Manic episode

        a) Period of at least 1 week during which mood is abnormally and persistently elevated, expansive, or irritated

        b) At least 3 of the following symptoms (if irritable, 4):

           (1) Inflated self-esteem or grandiose behavior

           (2) Decreased need for sleep

           (3) Unusual talkativeness

           (4) Flight of ideas or feeling that thoughts are racing

           (5) Easy distractibility

           (6) Increase in goal-directed activity or psychomotor agitation

           (7) Excessive involvement in activities that give pleasure but carry a high risk

        c) May range from mild to severe, with or without delusions or hallucinations

        d) Includes impairment that affects social and work lives

        e) May require hospitalization to prevent harm to self or others

2. Hypomanic episode
   a) Period of 4 days during which mood is sustained at elevated, expansive, or irritable levels
   b) Symptoms (same as section I,D,1,b of this chapter)
   c) Behavior obviously uncharacteristic of person
   d) Not as severe as manic episode (no psychotic features and does not cause marked impairment of work and social lives)
3. Cyclothymic disorder
   a) Numerous periods of hypomanic symptoms and of depressed mood or loss of pleasure for at least 2 years (1 year for children and adolescents)
   b) Occurs more than 2 months at a time
   c) No evidence of manic episode or major depressive episode
4. Possible configurations of bipolar disorders
   a) Manic episodes may occur alternately with major depressive episodes.
   b) Manic and major depressive episodes may occur together or may be mixed: Every day for at least 1 week, symptomatic behaviors of a major depressive episode and a manic episode exist.
   c) A single manic episode can occur without a major depressive episode.

E. Additional mood disorder categories (DSM-IV)
   1. Mood disorder due to a general medical condition
   2. Substance-induced mood disorder
   3. Mood disorder not otherwise specified

F. Theories of causation of mood disorders (usually involves a combination of factors)
   1. Psychophysiologic theories
      a) Genetics
         (1) Evidence suggests a genetically inherited susceptibility to mood disorders.
         (2) The precise role of genetics, however, is still unclear.
      b) Biologic model: emphasizes biochemical factors, including imbalances in neurotransmitters, hormones, and biologic rhythms as well as effects of medications and electroconvulsive therapy (ECT) on neurotransmitters.
   2. Psychoanalytic theories
      a) Anger turned inward: Aggression that is not able to be directed at the causative object is turned upon the self, causing depression.
      b) Object loss theory
         (1) Attributes depression to loss of a significant object of attachment
         (2) Assumes that the loss of a mother figure during childhood fol-lowed by a second significant loss in adulthood (e.g., significant person, job, marriage) becomes a triggering factor for depression
   3. Personality organization theory
      a) Suggests that low self-esteem causes depression and/or overcompensation (mania)

        b) Identifies 3 personality structures that predispose to depression
           (1) Dominant other: A person relies on another for self-esteem; the dependent person is clinging, passive, manipulative, and not goal-oriented.
           (2) Dominant goal: A person has an unrealistic goal and will not be happy unless it is achieved; the person becomes secretive, obsessive, and arrogant and engages in extensive wishful thinking and introspection.
           (3) Constant mode of feeling, or depressive character: A person has no goals; the person is often harsh and hypercritical and does not form meaningful relationships.
    4. Cognitive model
        a) Holds that depression occurs because of how the client evaluates the self and the environment
        b) Focuses on disturbed thinking (cognition) as the cause and disturbed affect as the result, which is the reverse of views held by other theories
    5. Learned helplessness model
        a) Holds that mood disorders result from a belief that one has no control over one's life or what happens
        b) Suggests that people resistant to depression have experienced mastery in their lives (i.e., they have experienced situations in which their actions exerted a meaningful influence over events or outcomes)
    6. Behavioral model
        a) Assumes that mood disturbances are learned
        b) Suggests that causes of a client's depression can be found in past patterns of behavior and interaction with the environment
        c) Suggests that depressive behaviors have occurred in the past owing to a lack of positive reinforcement or to punishing events (e.g., marital or job problems)
        d) Treatment aimed at increasing number of positive interactions and reinforcing events (e.g., by improving the client's social skills)

  G. Precipitating factors (factors that may trigger an episode of mood disturbance)
    1. Loss of attachment (e.g., loss of a significant other, status, self-esteem)
    2. Major life events or changes in role (e.g., graduation, job, marriage, parenthood [including postpartum depression occurring within 4 weeks of delivery])
    3. Lack of coping resources such as an extended family, friends, or income
    4. Physiologic changes (e.g., those associated with aging, medications, medical condition)

5. Substance abuse (e.g., alcohol, amphetamines, cocaine, sedative-hypnotics, opioids)
6. Time of year (associated with seasonal pattern)

II. Treatments

See text pages

A. Nondrug treatments
   1. Psychotherapy
   2. Behavioral therapy
   3. Cognitive therapy
   4. Family therapy
   5. Group therapy
   6. Relaxation therapy

B. Antidepressant medications
   1. Tricyclic antidepressants
      a) Examples: amitriptyline hydrochloride (Elavil, Endep), amoxapine (Asendin), imipramine hydrochloride (Tofranil)
      b) Benefits
         (1) Effective for acute and long-term depressive illness
         (2) Helps approximately 70% of people with acute depressive disorder
         (3) Commonly takes effect 1–3 weeks after therapy is begun; may take as long as 4–6 weeks
      c) Risks and cautions
         (1) Dry mouth, grogginess, weight gain, blurred vision, constipation, postural hypotension, urinary retention (especially in elderly clients), nausea, sweating, temporary confusion, speech blockage
         (2) Serious cardiac concerns: arrhythmias, tachycardia, myocardial infarction
         (3) May trigger seizure activity in susceptible individuals
         (4) Drug interactions: MAOIs, phenothiazines, alcohol, barbiturates, anticoagulants
         (5) Withdrawal symptoms caused by stopping suddenly
         (6) Overdose considerations (see Nurse Alert, "Signs of Tricyclic Overdose")
   2. Nontricyclic antidepressants (also called second-generation or atypical antidepressants)
      a) Examples: maprotiline (Ludiomil); fluoxetine hydrochloride (Prozac)
      b) Benefits
         (1) May be used when client does not respond to tricyclics
         (2) Fewer side effects (including cardiac) than tricyclics and faster onset of action
      c) Risks and cautions: persistent penile erection, nausea, tremors, grogginess, nervousness, insomnia, weight loss, dizziness
   3. Monoamine oxidase inhibitors (MAOIs)
      a) Examples: isocarboxazid (Marplan), phenelzine sulfate (Nardil)
      b) Benefits: effective antidepressants for clients who do not respond to tricyclics or nontricyclics

    c) Risks and cautions

        (1) Side effects greater than for tricyclics and nontricyclics

        (2) Risk of hypertensive crisis (may be triggered by certain foods) (see Nurse Alert, "Signs of Hypertensive Crisis with the Use of MAOIs," and Client Teaching Checklist, "Substances Contraindicated When Using MAOIs")

C. Electroconvulsive therapy (ECT) for depression (see Chapter 3, section VIII,A)

D. Antimania medications

    1. Lithium

        a) Types

            (1) Lithium carbonate (Eskalith, Lithotabs)

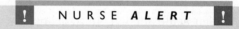

! NURSE *ALERT* !

Signs of Tricyclic Overdose

Potential for overdose of tricyclic antidepressants is high because all depressed clients have suicide risk potential.

Precautions:
- Only a 1-week supply should be given to a severely depressed client, whether suicidal or not. (Fatal dose of tricyclics is 10–30 times the daily dose [1000–3000 mg].)
- Check mouth of inpatient to be sure that each dose is swallowed as it is administered.

Early signs:
- Confusion
- Inability to concentrate
- Visual hallucinations

Overdose symptoms:
- Delirium
- Hyperthermia
- Convulsions
- Arrhythmias
- Coma
- Shock
- Respiratory failure

Actions:
- Report any symptoms to the physician.
- Induce emesis.
- Empty stomach with gastric lavage.
- Maintain airway.
- Maintain pulmonary function.

Signs of Hypertensive Crisis with the Use of MAOIs

Warning signs of hypertensive crisis:
- Increase in blood pressure
- Headache
- Heart palpitations

Symptoms of hypertensive crisis:
- Sudden, severe occipital headache radiating frontally
- Extreme rise in blood pressure
- Flushing of head and face
- Chest pain
- Sweating
- Nausea
- Vomiting
- Dilated pupils and photophobia
- Intracranial bleeding

Emergency treatment for hypertensive crisis:
- Notify physician immediately.
- Discontinue MAOIs.
- Keep client in upright position. (Lying down increases intracranial pressure.)
- Chlorpromazine, 100 mg, is administered intramuscularly as ordered.
- Phentolamine is administered slowly in doses of 5 mg intravenously as ordered.
- Reduce fever with use of ice packs, sponging, cold compresses, or bath of room-temperature water. Do not cover client if he/she has chills with fever.

        (2) Lithium carbonate, sustained-release (Lithobid, Eskalith CR)

        (3) Lithium citrate (Cibalith-S, Lithonate-S)

   b) Benefits: Lithium is the most often chosen medication for the manic phase of bipolar disorder; it may also be effective for other psychiatric conditions, such as bulimia, aggression, and schizophrenia.

   c) Risks and cautions

        (1) Possibility of increase in blood levels of lithium beyond therapeutic limit

           (a) Causes of increase in lithium levels

              i) Reduced sodium intake

              ii) Renal function impairment

              iii) Conditions leading to fluid and electrolyte imbalance (e.g., sweating, fever, vomiting)

           (b) Prevention measures: Divide doses or use timed-release capsules, monitor blood lithium levels, and monitor sodium and fluid intake and renal function (see Nurse Alert, "Monitoring Blood Lithium Levels," and Client Teaching Checklist, "Preventing Lithium Toxicity").

        (2) Overdose considerations

           (a) Signs of overdose: nausea, tremors, lethargy, dysarthria, hyperactive deep tendon reflexes, ataxia, tinnitus, vertigo, weakness, drowsiness

           (b) Effects of overdose: renal damage, circulatory damage, death

           (c) Requires immediate notification of physician

    2. Anticonvulsants

      a) Types: carbamazepine (Tegretol), valproic acid (Depakene), clonazepam (Klonopin)

      b) Uses: for mood stabilization when lithium is ineffective or contraindicated; for specific situations such as treatment of acute mania and prevention of manic episodes

✔ CLIENT TEACHING CHECKLIST ✔

Substances Contraindicated When Using MAOIs

Clients taking monoamine oxidase inhibitors (MAOIs) must be cautious about ingesting foods, liquids, or medications containing the amino acid tyramine. MAOIs block enzymes in the stomach that neutralize tyramine. As a result, large amounts of tyramine may reach the nerve cells that help control blood pressure, causing a hypertensive crisis. This dangerously high blood pressure can cause a stroke, aneurysms, heart failure, or even death.

In general, tyramines are found in food that is fermented, aged, pickled, smoked, or spoiled. Teach the client to avoid these substances:

✔ Aged or processed cheeses
✔ Aged, pickled, or smoked meats, poultry, or fish
✔ Beer, red wine, liquor, and sherry
✔ Yeast
✔ Fava beans
✔ Liver (especially chicken)
✔ Overripe fruit, such as bananas
✔ Raisins
✔ Yogurt
✔ Soy sauce
✔ Cold medications, antihistamines, and decongestants
✔ Narcotics (e.g., cocaine)
✔ Asthma inhalants
✔ Caffeine (e.g., colas, tea, coffee)
✔ Epinephrine, including local anesthetics that contain it
✔ Amphetamines and diet pills
✔ Other medications, both prescription and over-the-counter, unless approved by a physician

III. Essential nursing care

A. Nursing assessment
1. Record observations of client's behavior and affect.
2. Assess responses.
    a) Physical reactions
    b) Behavioral responses
    c) Affective responses
    d) Cognitive responses
3. Collect data to differentiate between mood disorders and physical and other psychiatric disorders that produce symptoms resembling mood disorders (e.g., organic mental disease mimicking depression, panic mimicking mania).
4. Use assessment tools to determine the extent or degree of depression or mania (e.g., Beck Depression Inventory, Zung Self-Rating Depression Scale, Manic-State Rating Scale).
5. Assess potential of client to harm self or others (see Nurse Alert, "Identifying the Client at Risk for Suicide").

See text pages
_____

B. Nursing diagnoses
    1. Main NANDA nursing diagnoses
        a) Potential for violence, self-directed or directed at others
        b) Potential for injury
        c) Altered thought processes
        d) Dysfunctional grieving
        e) Hopelessness
        f) Powerlessness
    2. Additional NANDA nursing diagnoses
        a) Ineffective individual coping
        b) Spiritual distress (distress of the human spirit)
        c) Anxiety
        d) Self-esteem disturbance
        e) Impaired social interaction
        f) Altered nutrition
        g) Self-care deficits

Zung Self-Rating Depression Scale*

	None or Little of the Time	Some of the Time	A Good Part of the Time	Most or All of the Time
1. I feel down-hearted, blue and sad	1	2	3	4
2. Morning is when I feel the best	4	3	2	1
3. I have crying spells or feel like it	1	2	3	4
4. I have trouble sleeping through the night	1	2	3	4
5. I eat as much as I used to	4	3	2	1
6. I enjoy looking at, talking to and being with attractive women/men	4	3	2	1
7. I notice that I am losing weight	1	2	3	4
8. I have trouble with constipation	1	2	3	4
9. My heart beats faster than usual	1	2	3	4
10. I get tired for no reason	1	2	3	4
11. My mind is as clear as it used to be	4	3	2	1
12. I find it easy to do the things I used to do	4	3	2	1
13. I am restless and can't keep still	1	2	3	4
14. I feel hopeful about the future	4	3	2	1
15. I am more irritable than usual	1	2	3	4
16. I find it easy to make decisions	4	3	2	1
17. I feel that I am useful and needed	4	3	2	1
18. My life is pretty full	4	3	2	1
19. I feel that others would be better off if I were dead	1	2	3	4
20. I still enjoy the things I used to do	4	3	2	1

*A raw score of 50 or above is associated with depression requiring hospital treatment.

SOURCE: Zung, W. K. 1965. Zung self-rating depression scale. *Archives of General Psychiatry* 12:63–70. Copyright © 1965, American Medical Association.

Figure 7–1
Zung Self-Rating Depression Scale

NURSE *ALERT*

Identifying the Client at Risk for Suicide

Often suicide is associated with depression, but the client may also be at risk during a manic phase. Clients who experience command auditory hallucinations are also at risk and should be identified. Furthermore, the risk of suicide may increase as depressive symptoms improve, since clients may become goal-directed enough to formulate and carry out a suicide plan.

Assessment rating scales can help health care providers identify clients at risk. In addition, key warning signs of the client at risk include:

- Remarks such as, "Will you remember me when I'm gone?"
- Lack of plans or concern about the future or canceling plans
- Putting one's affairs in order, such as making a will or funeral arrangements
- Giving away valuable or cherished belongings
- Withdrawal from friends and social relationships
- Evidence of a specific, feasible suicide plan and the means to carry it out
- Inability to concentrate or to sleep (sleep deprivation)
- Apparent sudden recovery from depression

If you believe a client might be contemplating suicide, ask the person if she/he has ever thought about harming herself/himself. Research has found that asking about suicide will not provoke an attempt and may lessen the person's anxiety.

      h) Sexual dysfunction
      i) Sleep pattern disturbance
      j) Altered family processes
  3. Selected complete nursing diagnoses
      a) Ineffective individual coping related to spouse's death evidenced by statements indicating fear of living alone
      b) Potential for injury related to manic episodes evidenced by history of recent auto accidents

C. Planning (goal setting)
  1. General goals
      a) Assist client in developing coping mechanisms.
      b) For normal grief reactions, reassure client that feelings are normal, and help ensure that the grieving process is completed.
      c) For unresolved grief reactions, help client reinitiate and complete all stages of the normal grieving process.
      d) Promote and support client's recognition and expression of feelings.
      e) Promote client's self-esteem.
      f) Promote client's insight and ability to identify stressors.
      g) Promote client's interpersonal relationships.
  2. Examples of specific goals
      a) Client will express acceptance of his/her loss at the conclusion of the mourning process.

       b) Client will be able to identify places or people to contact if suicidal thoughts occur.

       c) Client will be able to concentrate on a specific task for a reasonable length of time.

D. Nursing implementation (intervention)
1. General interventions for any mood disorder
    a) Provide emotional support for client and family.
    b) Project sense of confidence and control, a sense that you can help the client.
    c) Provide for client's safety.
    d) Address client's physical well-being.
       (1) Monitor diet and nutritional status.
       (2) Plan activities appropriate to client's energy level.
       (3) Promote healthy sleep and rest habits.
          (a) Provide rest periods if necessary, but discourage napping or staying in bed, since they may interfere with sleeping patterns at night.
          (b) Provide education about and interventions for insomnia, such as baths, massage, and soft music.
          (c) Encourage client to reduce caffeine consumption, especially late in the day.
       (4) Offer positive reinforcement when client takes responsibility for self-care.
    e) Establish contracts with client regarding impulse control and self-care.
       (1) Establish "no running" contract, in which client agrees to confront issues rather than withdraw from them.
       (2) Establish "no secrets" contract, in which client agrees to work openly and honestly with the therapeutic team.
       (3) If necessary, establish "no suicide, no homicide" contract, in which client agrees not to harm self or others.
    f) Use the "pace and lead" intervention for clients with excessive or deficient affect or behavior.
       (1) Pacing is matching one's pace (e.g., rate of talking, behavior) to that of the client.
       (2) Leading, which occurs after pacing, is changing one's pace (faster or slower) to promote changes in the client's affect or behavior.
    g) Assist client in establishing structure through the use of scheduled activities, behavioral contracts, and recording of daily activities, behaviors, and emotions.
    h) Teach relaxation techniques to the client (see Chapter 5, section II,C).

i) Actively listen to the client.

j) Employ empathy.

k) Offer positive reinforcement for healthy behavior.

l) Administer medications as ordered, and monitor drug effects.

    (1) For postural hypotension, assess for risk of falls, take vital signs while client is standing and sitting, explain to client that he/she may feel dizzy, and instruct client to rise slowly from bed or chair to prevent dizziness or blackouts.

    (2) For anticholinergic effects of antidepressants (dry mouth, blurred vision, constipation, urinary retention, sweating), provide fluids, and caution client about driving and use of machinery.

    (3) For cardiac concerns, assess cardiac function if indicated by history or orders.

2. Interventions for grief reactions

a) Develop one's own self-awareness through examination of losses in one's past and related feelings.

b) Offer anticipatory guidance, if possible.

    (1) Help client understand the grieving process before the loss occurs.

    (2) Provide opportunities for client to express feelings and thoughts about the impending loss.

c) Assist in grief work.

d) Provide opportunity for grieving as well as settings in which it may take place.

e) Recognize expressions of hostility toward the staff as part of the bereavement process.

f) Assist client in obtaining additional emotional support from his/her social network (e.g., family, friends, clergy, social agencies).

g) Identify those at risk for delayed or prolonged grief reactions.

h) Recognize that termination of the nurse-client relationship, while necessary, also involves a loss to the client; provide time to explore those feelings.

3. Interventions for depression

a) Implement measures to prevent suicide if client is at risk.

    (1) Notify physician of risk factors.

    (2) Provide for continuous monitoring.

    (3) Provide reassurance to the client that he/she will not be permitted to harm self.

b) Adopt warm, accepting approach for depressed clients, recognizing that they may resist attempts to establish a therapeutic relationship.

c) Avoid attempts to "cheer up" the depressed client.

d) Acknowledge and accept the client's feelings, but do not sympathize or identify with those feelings; establish a calm, confident, and objective manner.

e) Express hope to the client.

f) Encourage client to express thoughts and emotions, including negative emotions (which are typically blocked in depression).

g) Provide cognitive interventions.
   (1) Help the client develop a sense of control over goals and behavior.
   (2) Increase the client's self-esteem by helping client modify negative expectations.

h) Provide behavioral interventions; implement them gradually.
   (1) Promote successful, goal-oriented behavior.
   (2) Redirect the client away from inwardly directed behaviors (e.g., introspection, passive behavior) to outwardly directed behavior (e.g., social interaction).
   (3) Provide structured activities, beginning with short-duration activities with a high likelihood of being performed successfully.
   (4) Provide positive reinforcement for desired behavior.

i) Provide social interventions.
   (1) Spend time with the client to establish rapport.
   (2) Teach and model effective social skills.
   (3) Employ role-playing techniques, rehearsal, feedback, and positive reinforcement for adaptive social skills.
   (4) Provide opportunities for the client to practice and refine skills.
   (5) Help client identify social organizations and groups through which the client can expand his/her social network.
   (6) Involve the family in the client's therapy and discharge planning; provide family education and counseling.
   (7) Educate client about drug effects: Explain that symptoms may not begin to improve for a week or more.

j) Take measures to prevent MAOI interactions in clients taking these drugs (see Nurse Alert, "Signs of Hypertensive Crisis with the Use of MAOIs," and Client Teaching Checklist, "Substances Contraindicated When Using MAOIs").

4. Interventions for mania
   a) Implement precautions against accidents or destructive episodes.
   b) Maintain consistent and well-structured care plan.
   c) Ensure that client attends to basic physical needs (e.g., eating, sleeping, hygiene).
   d) Avoid group activities for extremely manic client, especially activities involving competition.
   e) Provide clear, concise instruction.
   f) Recognizing that the client may engage in manipulative behavior and may resist therapy, be calm yet firm.
   g) Monitor intake and output, particularly of fluids and sodium. (See section II,D,1 of this chapter for effects of lithium.)

h) Review client's impact on the nursing staff (e.g., feelings of conflict, resentment, and defensiveness related to the client's behavior).

E. Nursing evaluation
   1. Review goals, and assess progress.
      a) Client demonstrates reduction in or elimination of suicidal or hostile thoughts.
      b) Client demonstrates improved self-care.
      c) Client resumes some social activities.
      d) Client's self-esteem increases.
      e) Client shows improvement in ability to concentrate.
      f) Client and family understand information about medication, including facts about overdose and side effects.
   2. If goals were not achieved, assess reasons.
      a) Were goals realistic?
      b) Were problems identified correctly?
      c) Was enough time allowed to achieve goals?
   3. Revise goals and care plan as necessary.

1. Ms. Martino is admitted to the inpatient psychiatric unit with a diagnosis of major depression. Her depressive symptoms, which began 1 month ago, include anorexia with a 10-lb weight loss, excessive sleep, and difficulty in completing activities of daily living. She is withdrawn and preoccupied with her thoughts. Which of Ms. Martino's needs should the nurse address first?

   a. Hygiene activities
   b. Socialization
   c. Nutritional habits
   d. Sleep habits

2. During the first week of treatment, Ms. Martino is most likely to respond to which nursing intervention?

   a. Helping the client choose a recreational activity
   b. Offering the client reading material about depression
   c. Having the client reminisce about a happy event
   d. Assisting the client with self-care

3. An appropriate nursing diagnosis for a client receiving tricyclic antidepressants would be:

   a. Potential for fluid volume deficit related to diuretic effects of medication.
   b. Constipation related to anticholinergic effects of medication.
   c. Urge incontinence related to cholinergic effects of medication.
   d. Ineffective breathing patterns related to CNS depressant effects of medication.

4. When utilizing a cognitive framework, the nurse encourages a depressed client to:

   a. Explore childhood memories.
   b. Identify negative thoughts and develop alternative ideas.
   c. Recognize feelings of loss of control.
   d. Identify learned negative behaviors.

5. A client who is being treated for depression is receiving the second-generation anti-depressant trazodone hydrochloride (Desyrel) 50 mg TID. She complains of feeling dizzy after taking her medication. The nurse should first:

   a. Withhold the trazodone hydrochloride, and notify the physician.
   b. Administer future doses with meals.
   c. Consult the physician for a dosage reduction.
   d. Increase the client's fluid intake to 2000 ml per day.

6. Client teaching for a client taking phenelzine sulfate (Nardil), a monoamine oxidase inhibitor (MAOI), includes the instruction to:

   a. Avoid aged cheeses and pickled meats.
   b. Stay out of the sun, since the skin is photosensitive.
   c. Have blood pressure taken daily.
   d. Monitor weight, since weight loss may occur.

7. Susan, age 35, is admitted to the inpatient psychiatric unit with a diagnosis of bipolar disorder, manic phase. She is hyperactive and intrusive; her speech is rapid and pressured. She moves continually around the unit. At mealtime, Susan says, "No lunch for me. I've got too much to do." The most appropriate nursing intervention at this time would be to:

   a. Recognize that Susan will eat when she is hungry.
   b. Provide a tray for Susan, and redirect her to her room.
   c. Remind Susan that she will be restricted to the unit until she begins eating.
   d. Offer Susan high-calorie finger foods that she can eat while she is active.

8. During the nursing assessment, Susan tells the nurse that she is going to start her own business, that she just returned from a trip to Europe, and that she would like to rearrange her hospital room. The nurse recognizes this rapid shifting of topics as:
   a. Flight of ideas.
   b. Perseveration.
   c. Pressured speech.
   d. Loose associations.

9. Susan is started on lithium carbonate, 300 mg 3 times a day. Which of the following does the nurse recognize as a risk factor for developing lithium toxicity?
   a. Increased blood pressure
   b. Vomiting and diarrhea
   c. Weight gain
   d. Sustained salt intake

10. Which observation by the nurse would be most expected in a client with hypomanic episode of bipolar disorder?
    a. The client exhibits delusional thinking.
    b. The client expresses feelings of helplessness and insecurity.
    c. The client is in a sustained elevated mood.
    d. The client sleeps excessively and complains of fatigue.

11. Which nursing action is most effective for the client in an acute manic state?
    a. Talking to the client about his/her feelings
    b. Reducing the opportunity for stimulation
    c. Having the client participate in group activities
    d. Teaching the client role-playing techniques

12. When assessing a client for side effects of treatment with lithium carbonate, the nurse is most likely to observe which of the following responses?
    a. Fine hand tremor
    b. Persistent stomach upset
    c. Ataxia
    d. Slurred speech

ANSWERS

1. **Correct answer is c.** Basic nutritional needs are of primary concern for this client because she has had a 10-lb weight loss and may also be dehydrated.

   a. Hygiene needs can be addressed gradually.
   b. Socialization can be addressed as the client improves.
   d. Excessive sleeping may continue until antidepressant therapy begins to take effect.

2. **Correct answer is d.** The client will most likely respond to efforts by the nurse to structure time to assist her with self-care needs. This is a supportive intervention by which the nurse demonstrates concern and helps to motivate the client.

   a. A recreational activity is not appropriate for a client who has low energy. It serves to focus the client's attention on her lack of energy and interest. As her mood improves, a recreational activity will help her to become active.
   b. Depressed clients are usually unable to concentrate on reading materials.
   c. Reminiscing about a happy event may be appropriate later in the client's treatment. During the first week of treatment, the client is not likely to be able to recall a happy event. It is typical of depression for thoughts to be negative and hopeless.

3. **Correct answer is b.** Tricyclic antidepressants (TCAs) have anticholinergic side effects, which include constipation.

   a. TCAs have no diuretic effects.
   c. TCAs have anticholinergic side effects. Urinary retention, not urge incontinence, would be expected.
   d. TCAs do not have respiratory depressant effects.

4. **Correct answer is b.** Cognitive approaches focus on thought processes.

   a. Exploring childhood memories is indicative of a psychoanalytic approach.

c. Recognizing feelings of loss of control is associated with the theory of learned helplessness.

d. Behavioral models focus on learned behaviors.

5. **Correct answer is b.** Administering trazodone hydrochloride (Desyrel) with meals or at bedtime minimizes the dizziness and sedation that may occur as side effects.

a. Dizziness is a common side effect, not a sign of toxicity. There is no reason to withhold the drug when the symptom can probably be managed with appropriate interventions.

c. If the dizziness is too distressing for the client and if taking trazodone hydrochloride with meals does not help, dosage reduction would be appropriate. However, it is not the best initial choice.

d. Dizziness due to trazodone hydrochloride is related to central nervous system (CNS) effects, not fluid imbalance. Forcing fluid intake is unlikely to relieve it.

6. **Correct answer is a.** Use of MAOIs requires dietary restrictions on foods high in tyramine. MAOIs inhibit the action of monoamine oxidase, which is an enzyme responsible for breaking down tyramine in dietary sources. Common categories of foods high in tyramine are aged cheeses and pickled meats.

b. Skin sensitivity is not a side effect of MAOIs.

c. Orthostatic hypotension may occur, as with any antidepressant; however, taking daily blood pressures is not indicated. Hypertensive crisis may occur as a result of combining an MAOI with a tyramine-rich food; however, this is managed with dietary restrictions, not with daily blood pressure measurement.

d. Weight gain, not loss, is a likely side effect of an MAOI.

7. **Correct answer is d.** The nurse recognizes the priority need of nutrition and utilizes an approach that will be useful for the client. In this hyperactive state, the client is most likely to be receptive to food that she can eat easily without unnecessary restrictions.

a. Relying on the client to eat when she is hungry is inappropriate, because in a hyperactive state, she can easily become dehydrated and nutritionally compromised.

b. Because Susan's judgment and behavior control are poor, it is unlikely that she will be able to eat without supervision by the nurse.

c. Restricting the client to the unit until she eats is a behavioral technique that will be effective later in Susan's treatment. While she is acutely manic, it is unlikely that she could respond to this type of intervention.

8. **Correct answer is a.** Flight of ideas is commonly seen in a manic client. The client jumps from topic to topic in a nearly continuous flow of speech.

b. Perseveration is the involuntary repetition of the same thought, phrase, or motor response to different questions or situations. It is associated with organic brain disorders.

c. Pressured speech is the quality or tone of speech observed in the manic client. It is a forceful, driven type of speech that frequently accompanies flight of ideas.

d. Loose associations is the illogical stream of thoughts or ideas seen most frequently in schizophrenic disorders.

9. **Correct answer is b.** Vomiting and diarrhea may lead to dehydration, which can cause lithium to rise to toxic blood levels.

a. Changes in blood pressure do not effect lithium levels.

c. Weight gain commonly occurs with lithium use and does not indicate that toxicity may occur.

d. Constant level of normal salt intake is recommended for clients taking lithium. Since lithium decreases sodium reabsorption by the renal tubules, it could lead to sodium depletion. A low sodium intake causes a relative increase in lithium retention, which could lead to toxicity.

10. **Correct answer is c.** Elevated mood in the absence of impaired reality testing is an indication of hypomania.

    a. Delusional thoughts that impair reality testing are not present in hypomania.
    b. Clients with a diagnosis of hypomania are likely to exaggerate their ability.
    d. Clients with a diagnosis of hypomania are more likely to have difficulty sleeping due to their elevated mood.

11. **Correct answer is b.** Minimizing stimulation during the manic phase of illness helps diminish hyperactivity.

    a. Clients who are diagnosed with mania are not able to focus on their inner feelings in a productive, introspective manner. Behavior control is the focus of treatment in the acute phase of mania.

    c. Group activities are not recommended for clients with a diagnosis of mania, because of the stimulation of the group setting.
    d. Role-playing is a technique that requires abstract thought. This is not effective for clients who are hyperactive and very distractible.

12. **Correct answer is a.** Fine hand tremor is an expected side effect which usually subsides with treatment.

    b. Mild nausea may occur initially but also subsides with treatment. Persistent stomach upset is a sign of advanced lithium toxicity.
    c. Ataxia is a sign of severe lithium toxicity.
    d. Slurred speech is an early sign of lithium toxicity.

8

Cognitive Disorders

NURSING HIGHLIGHTS

1. The types of cognitive disorders most frequently encountered by nurses are delirium and dementia.
2. Nursing care for both delirium and dementia is supportive and is aimed at keeping the client oriented to time, space, and person.
3. Nurse should protect the client with delirium or dementia from harm and should address physical needs such as hygiene and skin integrity.
4. Goals set by the nurse in the care plan should be realistic, based on client's specific diagnosis, level of functioning, and prospects for improvement or maintenance.
5. Educating family members about dementia, its likely progression, and community resources can help them cope with the long-term care of loved ones.

agnosia—inability to recognize objects or to grasp the meaning of words, objects, or symbols

aphasia—loss of language ability; inability to remember correct name for an object or a person

apraxia—inability to perform purposeful movements

labile affect—unstable, changeable, uncontrolled expression of feelings or emotions

neuritic plaques—degenerating neuron material found in brain tissue of clients with Alzheimer's disease

neurofibrillary tangles—entwined filaments within a neuron; found mainly in the part of the brain responsible for short-term memory and emotion

pseudodementia—depression that mimics dementia

reality orientation—a nursing approach in which the client's orientation to time, place, and person is systematically reinforced

ENHANCED OUTLINE

I. General concepts

See text pages

A. DSM-IV changes in categorization
   1. The umbrella category of organic mental disorder (OMD), which was used in DSM-III-R to cover dementias, delirium, organic delusional syndrome, amnestic syndrome, organic hallucinations, organic mood syndrome, organic anxiety syndrome, organic personality syndrome, and intoxication and withdrawal due to psychoactive substance ingestion or stoppage, is *not* being used in DSM-IV to avoid giving the false impression that conditions not listed in DSM as OMDs do not have a biologic basis.
   2. Conditions listed in DSM-III-R as organic mental disorders are included in DSM-IV under the following categories:
      a) Delirium, dementia, amnestic, and other cognitive disorders
      b) Mental disorders due to a general medical condition: Disorders that may be related to a medical condition are listed in this section of DSM-IV but are discussed under the main section covering that disorder.
      c) Substance-related disorders (see Chapter 9 for material covered in this section of DSM-IV): This section of DSM-IV also lists specific disorders that are substance induced, but the diagnosis parameters of a disorder brought on by substance abuse are discussed under the main section covering that disorder (e.g., alcohol-induced mood disorder is discussed under mood disorders).

B. Definition
   1. Cognitive dysfunctions, or organic mental disorders, involve impairments of memory and of the ability to think and reason logically and effectively.
   2. Physical damage to or degeneration of the central nervous system (CNS) prevents the brain from accepting and processing information.

3. Cognitive impairment may result in disturbances of consciousness, rational and abstract thought, perception, judgment, memory, and language.
4. Cognitive impairment may be permanent or temporary, progressive or reversible, or mild or severe.

C. Causes of cognitive impairment
1. Toxins (e.g., heavy metals)
2. Trauma
3. Infection (e.g., HIV infection, encephalitis, pneumonia, brain infection)
4. Hypoxia (e.g., due to diminished blood flow caused by arteriosclerosis)
5. Metabolic disorders (e.g., hypothyroidism, hypoglycemia)
6. Lesions or tumors
7. Nutritional deficiencies (e.g., thiamine deficiencies, malnutrition)
8. Neurologic disease (e.g., Huntington's chorea)
9. Prescription drugs (e.g., digitalis, lithium, levodopa)
10. Nonprescription drugs (e.g., overmedication, drug reactions)
11. Postoperative states
12. Psychoactive substance abuse (e.g., cocaine use, alcoholism)
13. Psychosocial stressors (e.g., sensory deprivation, sensory overload, anxiety)

D. Treatments
1. If underlying medical conditions (e.g., infection, circulatory disorders) cause or contribute to the cognitive disorder, medical treatment is aimed at these conditions.
2. For some cognitive disorders, medical treatments are ineffective; therapy is aimed promoting optimal functioning, maintaining basic life skills and adequate nutrition as long as possible, and providing a safe environment and supportive care.
3. For delirium associated with withdrawal from alcohol or drugs, benzodiazepines, especially chlordiazepoxide (Librium), are used to treat withdrawal and to reduce anxiety.

See text pages

_____

II. Delirium: state of disturbed cognition caused by underlying medical condition or by substance intoxication or withdrawal

A. Characteristics
1. Rapid onset
2. Usually brief course (hours or days)
3. Usually reversible
4. Clouded consciousness
5. Disordered thought
6. Sensory misperceptions
7. Memory disturbance, especially concerning recent events
8. Fluctuating levels of awareness and intensity with some lucid periods during the day
9. Mood swings

    10. Generally worse at night and perhaps during early morning hours

    11. EEG changes

B. Typical behaviors
    1. Limited attention span
    2. Disturbed sleep-wake cycle
    3. Disorientation to time, place, and person
    4. Confusion
    5. Disturbing, usually visual, hallucinations
    6. Aggressive or destructive actions
    7. Expressions of fear and anxiety, perhaps followed by apathy
    8. Impulsive actions such as undressing at inappropriate times
    9. Agitation
    10 Restlessness
    11. Incoherence or slurred speech
    12. Changes in psychomotor activity

C. Types (DSM-IV)
    1. Delirium due to a general medical condition
    2. Substance-induced delirium
    3. Delirium due to multiple etiologies

D. Diagnostic criteria (DSM-IV)
    1. Reduced clarity of awareness of environment along with reduced ability to focus, sustain, or shift attention
    2. A change in cognition (e.g., memory deficit, disorientation, language disturbance, perceptual disturbance) that cannot be attributed to preexisting, established, or evolving dementia
    3. Development over a short time period (hours or days), usually varying during course of day
    4. Evidence produced through history, physical examination, and laboratory findings that there is a causal relationship to an underlying medical condition, to intoxication with or withdrawal from medications or other drugs, or to a combination of these conditions

E. Treatment: aimed at identifying and correcting underlying disorder, which may become irreversible and lead to dementia if untreated

III. Dementias: cognitive impairments that may be primary (not related to another disorder) or secondary (related to another medical condition or to a drug)

See text pages

A. Characteristics
    1. Usually gradual onset
    2. Progressive decline over months or years in the client's previous level of functioning
    3. May be irreversible
    4. No clouding of consciousness as in delirium
    5. Impaired abstract thinking
    6. Impaired judgment
    7. First short-term, then long-term memory impairment

8. Nonfluctuating symptoms
9. Personality changes (changes in person's usual personality or exaggeration of person's usual personality)
10. Usually no EEG changes
11. Most often affects the elderly (see Nurse Alert, "How to Differentiate between Dementia and Depression among the Elderly")

B. Typical behaviors
1. Anxiety during early stages, due to awareness that faculties are failing
2. Disorientation
3. Making up information to cover memory loss (confabulation)
4. Labile affect
5. Restlessness, especially at night
6. Agitation, especially as a resistance to change
7. Inappropriate social behavior (e.g., loss of inhibitions)

C. Types (DSM-IV)
1. Dementia of the Alzheimer's type (see section IV of this chapter)
2. Vascular dementia
3. Dementia due to other general medical conditions
4. Substance-induced persisting dementia
5. Dementia due to multiple etiologies

D. Diagnostic criteria (DSM-IV)
1. For all dementias
   a) Cognitive deficits that include both of the following:
      (1) Memory impairment: cannot learn new information and cannot remember previously learned information
      (2) At least 1 of the following cognitive disturbances:
         (a) Aphasia
         (b) Apraxia

! NURSE *ALERT* !

How to Differentiate between Dementia and Depression among the Elderly

Dementia
- Usually gradual onset of symptoms
- Attempts by client to cover up memory loss
- Anxiety about overcoming cognitive deficits
- Labile affect

Depression
- Time of onset usually more precisely identified than with dementia
- No attempt by client to hide memory loss
- Apathetic; doesn't try to remember
- Consistently depressed affect

NOTE: Depression may be present in a person who has dementia.

              (c) Agnosia

              (d) Inability to plan, organize, sequence, or abstract

      b) Significant impairment in social and occupational functioning

      c) Significant decline from former level of functioning

      d) Deficits not related exclusively to episodes of delirium

  2. Additional criteria for Alzheimer's dementia

      a) Gradual onset

          (1) Early onset: at age 65 or younger

          (2) Late onset: after age 65

      b) Continuing decline

      c) Cognitive deficits not due to CNS or systemic conditions or induced by substances

  3. Additional criteria for vascular dementia: neurologic signs (e.g., weak extremities, exaggerated deep tendon reflexes, gait abnormalities) and symptoms or laboratory evidence of cerebrovascular disease

  4. Additional criteria for dementia due to other general medical conditions: evidence from history, physical examination, or laboratory findings of 1 of the following conditions:

      a) HIV infection

      b) Head trauma

      c) Parkinson's disease

      d) Huntington's disease

      e) Pick's disease

      f) Creutzfeldt-Jakob disease

      g) Normal-pressure hydrocephalus

      h) Hypothyroidism

      i) Brain tumor

      j) Deficiency of vitamin B_{12}, folic acid, or niacin

      k) Neurosyphilis

  5. Additional criteria for substance-induced persisting dementia: evidence from history, physical examination, or laboratory findings of use of medication or toxins or of drugs being abused (e.g., inhalants, alcohol, sedative-hypnotics)

  6. Additional criteria for dementia due to multiple etiologies: evidence of a combination of causes (e.g., a general medical condition plus substance abuse)

E. Treatments

  1. For primary dementia, no effective medical treatments are known; care is aimed at maintaining optimal function.

  2. For secondary dementia, medical treatments are aimed at eliminating underlying cause.

IV. Alzheimer's disease

A. General concepts

  1. Alzheimer's disease is a form of primary dementia.

  2. It is the most commonly occurring type of dementia.

  3. The clinical course is progressive and irreversible, covering 1–10 years.

See text pages

B. Causes: The cause is unknown. Possible etiologies include the following.
1. Genetics
    a) Alzheimer's disease runs in families.
    b) Defect in chromosome 21 has been found in people with the disease.
2. A virus
3. Presence of high levels of aluminum in the brain
4. Reduced levels of the neurotransmitter acetylcholine
5. Accumulation of protein in the brain
6. Autoimmune defects
7. Decreased blood flow to the brain

C. Effects on the brain
1. The formation of neuritic plaques and neurofibrillary tangles as well as loss of specific nerve cells
2. Degeneration of associational areas of the brain
3. Disruptions of the neurotransmitters acetylcholine and serotonin

D. Symptoms
1. Early stage: forgetting names and appointments, misplacing things, loss of energy and drive, depression, irritability, difficulty handling everyday work or personal activities (e.g., balancing a checkbook), and attempts to hide forgetfulness
2. Moderate to severe stage: appearance of apparent cognitive defects; no recall of recent events or facts such as current address or current date, although long-term memory may be preserved; increasing difficulty understanding everyday events; becoming lost; wandering aimlessly; paranoia; restlessness at night; agitation; violence; increasing aphasia, apraxia, and agnosia
3. Late stage: severe disorientation; psychotic symptoms; severe agitation; confinement to bed; inability to participate in self-care; loss of ability to talk or walk; stupor; coma; death, usually caused by infection, malnutrition, or dehydration

E. Treatment: Tacrine (Cognex) was approved by the FDA in 1993—designed to provide symptom relief and to increase attention span in some clients with mild or moderate cases; in general, care is aimed at maintaining optimal function.

V. Essential nursing care for cognitive impairment

See text pages

_____

A. Nursing assessment
1. Take health history, including dietary habits, history of hearing or vision impairment, history of head trauma, medication and psychoactive substance use, and alcohol consumption.
2. Take family history.
3. Assess the following areas of client's functioning.
    a) Appearance
    b) Manner (e.g., degree of cooperativeness)

      c) Attitude (e.g., defensiveness)

      d) Communication

      e) Perception (e.g., sight, hearing, ability to recognize people and objects, presence of illusions or hallucinations)

      f) Level of consciousness (e.g., stupor, alertness)

      g) Motor activity (e.g., balance, coordination)

      h) Ability to perform activities of daily living

      i) Mood and affect

      j) Orientation to time, place, situation, and person

      k) Memory, including immediate, short-term, and long-term

      l) Abstract reasoning

      m) Calculations

      n) Judgment

  4. Assess coping mechanisms.

  5. Record observations of client's behavior and affect.

  6. Assess potential of client for harm to self or others.

B. Nursing diagnoses

  1. Main NANDA nursing diagnoses

      a) Altered thought processes

      b) Potential for injury

      c) Impaired verbal communication

  2. Additional NANDA nursing diagnoses

      a) Ineffective individual coping

      b) Self-esteem disturbance

      c) Altered role performance

      d) Self-care deficit

      e) Altered family processes

      f) Potential fluid volume deficit

      g) Impaired physical mobility

      h) Altered sensory perceptions

      i) Potential impaired skin integrity

      j) Sleep pattern disturbance

      k) Altered nutrition, less than body requirements

      l) Altered patterns of urinary elimination

      m) Bowel incontinence

  3. Selected complete nursing diagnoses

      a) Altered thought processes related to delirium evidenced by mistaking a stethoscope for a snake

      b) Impaired verbal communication related to aphasia evidenced by inability to name objects correctly

      c) Potential for injury related to decreased cognitive functioning evidenced by wandering from hospital floor

      d) Self-care deficit related to poor hygiene and poor nutrition evidenced by unkempt appearance and weight loss

C. Planning (goal setting)

  1. General goals

      a) Promote physiologic needs, including client safety and hygiene.

b) Promote optimal cognitive, memory, and perceptual functioning to enhance client's self-esteem and integrity.

c) Promote and support client's self-care activities.

d) When an underlying condition is a causative or contributing factor in cognitive impairment, assist in management of condition (e.g., provide care related to fever and decreased fluid intake associated with an infection that has produced delirium).

e) Promote family knowledge and skills in assisting client and in coping with client's condition.

2. Examples of specific goals for delirium
   a) Client will sleep 4–6 hours a night within 2 days.
   b) Client will demonstrate orientation to time, place, and person by the time of discharge from the hospital.
   c) Client will maintain adequate hydration.

3. Examples of specific goals for dementia
   a) Client will maintain appropriate level of physical activity.
   b) Client will reduce resistance to self-care measures.
   c) Client will wander only within prescribed areas.
   d) Client will wear ID information that cannot be removed to ensure safe return to hospital or home if he/she wanders away.
   e) Client's family will state that they are receiving emotional support from health care team.

D. Nursing implementation (intervention)
   1. Address client's physical well-being.
      a) Administer and monitor medications as ordered.
      b) Promote personal hygiene and grooming.
         (1) Monitor skin integrity and hygienic practices.
         (2) Provide assistance and step-by-step instructions as necessary.
         (3) Alter hygiene and grooming schedule to accommodate client's alertness phases.
         (4) Encourage client to do as much self-care as possible without assistance.
      c) Ensure adequate nutrition and hydration.
         (1) Monitor food intake.
         (2) Monitor fluid and electrolyte balance.
      d) Ensure physical safety.
         (1) Provide continuous observation during periods of agitation.
         (2) Ensure that the client's room does not contain objects that may hurt him/her.
         (3) Be sure that security measures are instituted to prevent wandering or inadvertent self-harm.
         (4) Identify potential causes of wandering (e.g., medication schedules, attention-seeking behavior, avoidance of stressful procedures), and seek to reduce or eliminate them.

(5) Use restraints only upon a physician's order, and provide continuous monitoring.
- e) Employ methods to promote needed rest and sleep.
  - (1) Provide methods of relaxation (e.g., back rubs, warm milk).
  - (2) Promote physical activity and socialization during the day (but do not overtax client).
2. Promote cognitive, memory, and perceptual functioning.
   - a) Continuously orient the client to time, place, situation, and person.
     - (1) Several times an hour if needed
     - (2) Especially at night, when disorientation is generally worse and client may be most frightened or upset
   - b) Keep client's room well lighted.
   - c) See that client has his/her eyeglasses, hearing aid, or other devices needed to assist perception.
   - d) Keep clock and calendar in view of the client.
   - e) If appropriate, use reality orientation techniques (i.e., systematically reinforcing the client's orientation to time, place, and person, usually in a group setting). (Clients with Alzheimer's disease who no longer recognize reality do not benefit from reality orientation.)
   - f) Elevate the head of the bed if possible; visual hallucinations are more likely if the client is flat on his/her back.
   - g) Encourage family visits and caregiving; ask family to bring in client's familiar personal belongings.
   - h) Assign the same personnel to the client as often as possible, to assist in orientation.
   - i) Do not test the client's memory or other cognitive abilities unless necessary.
   - j) Allow client as much control and decision making as he/she is capable of.
   - k) Learn client's interests and skills, and help client to use them as appropriate.
   - l) When client resists performing a needed action, stop for a short time and then try again.
3. Promote effective communication.
   - a) Provide clear messages and instructions; repeat them as necessary and with the same wording each time.
   - b) Place yourself directly in front of the client, and speak slowly.
   - c) Use gestures to supplement verbal expression.
   - d) Touch the client only with care and only after telling him/her that you are going to do it.
   - e) Incorporate orientation cues into conversation (e.g., "I am Mary Smith, your nurse"; "It's time for your morning exercises").
   - f) Limit choices offered to the client.
   - g) If a client becomes agitated during conversation, change the topic.
   - h) Speak firmly to an aggressive client; set limits.
   - i) Do not argue with client about illusions or hallucinations, but do not agree that they are real, and do not ask client to explain more about them; reinforce reality.

  j) Correct client's misperceptions with care.
  k) Take conversational cues from the topic the client initiates; this technique helps alleviate client's frustration over increasing forgetfulness.
  l) Make requests; do not demand. Questions that can be answered with a "yes" or "no" are preferred. Avoid power struggles.
  m) Allow client to express fears and anxiety.
4. Reinforce effective coping techniques.
  a) Do not openly confront or argue with client about his/her use of such coping techniques as denial, confabulation, hoarding of food, or repetitive behaviors or words.
  b) Identify sources of anxiety, and remove or lessen them to the extent possible.
5. Provide client and family education.
  a) When possible, provide explanations to the client regarding his/her condition.
  b) Provide education to family members about care; reinforce physician's explanations of causation and prognosis.
  c) For client with progressive dementia, review postdischarge needs such as medication and safety precautions; ensure that family is aware of community resources and knows when and where to seek assistance.

E. Nursing evaluation
1. Review goals, and continually assess progress.
  a) To extent possible, client becomes oriented to time, place, situation, and person.
  b) Client is functioning at optimal level for stage of condition.
  c) Client's physical well-being has been maintained.
  d) Client is involved in self-care to the extent possible.
  e) Family of client understands client's condition and participates in the client's care.
  f) For reversible cognitive impairment, client returns to previous level of functioning.
2. If goals were not achieved, assess reasons.
  a) Were the goals appropriate to the client's functional level and prognosis?
  b) Was the entire staff involved in setting goals and evaluating care?
3. Revise goals and care plan as necessary to accommodate client's needs (e.g., adjust care plan as cognitive functioning in person with progressive dementia worsens).

1. The client who has developed delirium is most likely to exhibit:

   a. Auditory hallucinations.
   b. Confusion that worsens at night.
   c. Drowsiness.
   d. Delusional thinking.

2. To help distinguish between delirium and the early stages of dementia, it is important for the nurse to assess for:

   a. Memory loss.
   b. Anxiety.
   c. Cognitive impairment.
   d. Impaired speech.

3. If Mr. Borland, a client diagnosed with dementia, has developed apraxia, the nurse would expect to observe that he:

   a. Uses words incorrectly.
   b. Puts his arms into the legs of his trousers while dressing.
   c. Does not recognize family members.
   d. Is unable to write his name.

4. Assessment findings for a client who has dementia differ from those for a client who has depression in that the client who has dementia:

   a. Frequently answers "I don't know" to questions.
   b. Refuses to attempt tasks.
   c. Tends to confabulate.
   d. Retains normal personality traits.

5. The nursing diagnosis with highest priority for a client who has delirium is:

   a. Hypothermia.
   b. High risk for violence.
   c. Pain.
   d. High risk for injury.

6. An appropriate goal for Ms. Carpenter, who has moderate Alzheimer's disease, would be that she:

   a. Independently performs self-care after appropriate teaching.
   b. Performs self-care if given step-by-step instructions.
   c. Remains oriented to person, place, and time until discharge.
   d. Recognizes friends and family members when they visit.

7. To help maintain orientation to reality in a client who has delirium, the nurse should:

   a. Elevate the head of the client's bed.
   b. Talk to the client constantly while providing care.
   c. Keep room lighting dim to avoid overstimulation.
   d. Keep the bedside table clear of equipment and belongings.

8. Mr. Ellis, who is delirious, has been calling his roommate by his son's name. The nurse enters the room and finds Mr. Ellis standing beside the roommate's bed with his fist raised, shouting, "I'm going to beat some respect into you." The nurse should first:

   a. Obtain help to put Mr. Ellis back in bed, and apply a soft restraint.
   b. Obtain help to put Mr. Ellis back in bed, and administer the prescribed sedative.
   c. Make eye contact but avoid touching Mr. Ellis, and state calmly, "You are not to hit him. Tell me how you feel."
   d. Grasp Mr. Ellis's raised arm firmly and say, "You are not to hit him. Come with me."

9. Ms. Symes, who has Alzheimer's disease, is capable of brushing her own teeth but refuses to do so when asked by the nurse. Which nursing action should be tried first?

   a. Set out the necessary equipment, and leave her alone.
   b. Place the toothbrush in her hand, and begin the movement for her.
   c. Leave for 15–20 minutes, then repeat the request.
   d. Make the request again, using different words.

1. **Correct answer is b.** Confusion is the hallmark of delirium. It often worsens at night and during the early morning; it may clear during the day.

   a. Visual and tactile hallucinations may occur in delirium. Auditory hallucinations are more common with schizophrenia or depression.
   c. Clients who have delirium usually do not experience drowsiness. They are more often restless, apprehensive, or agitated.
   d. Delusions are associated with psychiatric disorders such as schizophrenia. Clients experiencing delirium are more likely to suffer errors in perception, such as illusions or visual hallucinations.

2. **Correct answer is d.** Speech is seldom affected in the early stages of dementia. Slurred or disorganized speech is common in delirium.

   a. Short-term memory is impaired in both delirium and early dementia.
   b. Anxiety is a feature of both delirium and dementia. It may be 1 of the earliest signs of delirium, and it may occur in a client with a diagnosis of dementia as the client recognizes memory losses and difficulties in task performance.
   c. Cognitive impairments, such as disorientation, impaired judgment, and poor performance of tasks that depend on short-term memory, are common in both delirium and dementia.

3. **Correct answer is b.** Apraxia is defined as loss of purposeful movement. The client who has apraxia can no longer perform previously familiar tasks.

   a. Incorrect use of words is symptomatic of aphasia.
   c. Loss of recognition of familiar objects or individuals is symptomatic of severe agnosia.
   d. Inability to write is symptomatic of dysgraphia.

4. **Correct answer is c.** The client who has dementia will attempt to hide memory losses by confabulating. Clients who are depressed readily admit to memory loss.

   a and **b.** Apathy, with decreased effort to perform tasks and absence of efforts to recall the answers to questions, is typical of the client with a diagnosis of depression. Clients with a diagnosis of dementia struggle to perform but become frustrated and often provide "near-miss" answers to questions.
   d. Family members often report personality changes in both depressed and demented clients. The client who has dementia may become suspicious or angry, while the client who is depressed becomes sad or apathetic.

5. **Correct answer is d.** Impaired judgment and rapid shifts in affect place the client with a diagnosis of delirium at great risk for injury. The client may wander and fall, fail to call for assistance, or disrupt necessary medical equipment while experiencing illusions or hallucinations or while feeling apprehensive. Keeping the client safe will be the nurse's first priority.

   a. An increased metabolic rate is often associated with delirium. This would produce hyperthermia.
   b. While a client experiencing delirium might become aggressive and demonstrate violent behavior, this is less likely to be a problem than accidental injury. A calm, caring approach can usually minimize aggression.
   c. Pain may occur if the underlying cause of the delirium is a painful disorder. It is not universal, however, and would not take priority over safety.

6. **Correct answer is b.** Apraxia that occurs during the moderate stage of Alzheimer's disease would be mild and should not prevent self-care.

   a. Memory deficits are likely to make independent self-care at this stage impossible. Ms. Carpenter may forget what she is supposed to do or how to do it if no one is available to provide instructions.

c. Orientation is a goal that is appropriate for a client who has delirium. The client with moderate Alzheimer's disease is unlikely to remain oriented. Frequent reorientation, especially to place and time, will continue to be needed despite therapy.
d. Because a client with moderate Alzheimer's disease would still recognize family and friends, this would not be an appropriate goal.

7. **Correct answer is a.** Keeping the head of the bed elevated provides a more normal visual perspective of important environmental cues, reducing the probability of illusions.

    b. The ability of the client with a diagnosis of delirium to process information is limited. Communications should be kept short, simple, and concrete. Constant conversation may lead to confusion by exceeding the client's information-processing capabilities.
    c. The room should be kept well lighted at all times to improve the accuracy of perception of environmental stimuli. Dim light increases the client's risk of misperceiving objects in the room.
    d. Meaningful personal articles such as pictures or figurines from home provide comfort and support and are unlikely to be misperceived. Medical equipment is unfamiliar and may be misinterpreted, so it should be kept out of sight.

8. **Correct answer is c.** Limits must be clearly and calmly set. The client who has delirium often can respond to verbal controls.

Verbal limit setting should be attempted before imposing restraints. Clients with delirium are often easily distracted. Providing an alternate activity (e.g., conversation with the nurse) may distract Mr. Ellis.

a and **b.** Physical and chemical restraints are often unnecessary and should be used only if the client has documented inability to respond to verbal limit setting.
d. The nurse should not touch the agitated client, since he may misinterpret this as a threat and respond with defensive violence toward the nurse.

9. **Correct answer is c.** Because moods are labile in clients with a diagnosis of dementia, the client's response may be different a short time later. The memory losses of Alzheimer's disease may be used to advantage in this situation, since Ms. Symes is likely to have forgotten both the request and her response when the nurse returns.

    a. Ms. Symes has probably refused to brush her teeth because she cannot remember how. Leaving her alone with the equipment will not help.
    b. While the client is refusing to perform the task, she will not be receptive to help and may even interpret this as a physical threat and respond defensively.
    d. When a client with a diagnosis of dementia does not understand a request, it should be stated again in the exact same words. The client who does not understand will most likely make a comment that indicates a need for clarification or will look confused rather than refusing the request.

9

Psychoactive Substance Use Disorders

OVERVIEW

I. General concepts
A. Terms
B. Theories of causation
C. Groups at risk for substance abuse
D. Codependency
E. Multiple drug abuse
F. Nurses and substance abuse

II. Types of substances commonly abused
A. Alcohol
B. Amphetamines
C. Cannabis
D. Cocaine
E. Hallucinogens
F. Opioids
G. Phencyclidine
H. Antianxiety agents, sedatives, and hypnotics

III. Treatments
A. Substance abuse treatment centers
B. Psychotherapy
C. 12-step programs
D. Drug therapies

IV. Essential nursing care
A. Nursing assessment
B. Nursing diagnoses
C. Planning
D. Nursing implementation
E. Nursing evaluation

NURSING HIGHLIGHTS

1. Treatment and nursing care are usually complicated by clients' denial of the problem (e.g., negative consequences of abuse such as divorce or loss of employment are often attributed to other causes).
2. The transition from use to abuse often occurs gradually, making it difficult to identify abuse.
3. Nurse must understand that substance abuse is a disease, not a moral failing.
4. Nurse should emphasize to client that abstinence is almost always necessary for effective recovery.
5. Nurse must keep expectations for treatment success realistic, because the rate of treatment failures and relapse among clients suffering from substance abuse is high.
6. Although total abstinence is the goal, it is not often achieved; instead, strive for increasing periods of abstinence.

7. Nurses play a key role in efforts to prevent substance abuse through education of at-risk populations, especially adolescents.

GLOSSARY

dysarthria—difficulty in speaking as a result of an emotional or physical disorder (e.g., stammering, stuttering)
dyskinesia—an impairment of voluntary muscular movement
dysphoria—a mood characterized by sadness and depression
dystonia—an impairment of muscle tone
enable—make it possible for a person who abuses substances to continue the substance-abusing behavior (e.g., assuming the household responsibilities of the person who abuses substances)
euphoria—in substance abuse, an exaggerated and excessive sense of well-being
hyperpyrexia—an extremely high body temperature
hypersomnia—excessively deep and long periods of sleep
nystagmus—involuntary vertical or horizontal movements of the eyes
synesthesia—experiencing a particular sensory input in terms of another sense (e.g., experiencing sounds as colors)

ENHANCED OUTLINE

I. General concepts

See text pages
_____

A. Terms
    1. Abuse: recurrent misuse of a substance resulting in problems with employment, health, family, the legal system, or social relationships
    2. Dependence: recurrent misuse of a substance resulting in clinically significant health problems
      a) Physical dependence
         (1) Tolerance develops: The body requires increasing amounts of the substance to achieve the same effect.
         (2) Withdrawal occurs: The body undergoes a substance-specific physical reaction when the substance is discontinued.
      b) Psychologic dependence: a sense of craving or need for the drug
    3. Intoxication: The body undergoes a substance-specific group of reversible behavioral and physical changes.

B. Theories of causation
    1. Biologic theories: A biologic predisposition may exist that leads some people to abuse substances.
      a) Tendency toward substance abuse often runs in families.
      b) Biochemical abnormalities have been discovered.
         (1) People who abuse alcohol metabolize ethanol more efficiently than do nonabusers, resulting in higher tolerance for alcohol.

(2) People who abuse substances have an increased susceptibility to the pleasurable effects of the substances, resulting in increased substance use to achieve these effects.

2. Psychologic theories: Certain personality traits are associated with increased risk of substance abuse.
   a) Inadequate problem-solving skills
   b) Desire to escape or avoid problems
   c) Dominating and judgmental attitudes that mask self-doubt and passivity
   d) Insecurity
   e) Perception of own parents as emotionally cold
   f) Rebelliousness toward authority
   g) Difficulty forming intimate relationships
   h) Narcissism
   i) Weak superego
   j) Dependency tendencies

3. Sociocultural theories: Certain factors are associated with increased risk of substance abuse.
   a) Cultural pressure
   b) Peer pressure
   c) Stress
   d) Economic deprivation
   e) Easy access to substances

4. Family systems theories
   a) Adult children of 2 alcoholic parents have a 70% chance of becoming alcoholics.
   b) Certain factors are associated with increased risk of substance abuse.
      (1) Inability to separate from parents
      (2) Emotionally cold or distant parents
      (3) Family history of substance abuse (role modeling)

C. Groups at risk for substance abuse
   1. Adolescents
      a) Substance abuse among adolescents is widespread.
      b) Adolescents who abuse substances often have failed to complete a necessary developmental stage and remain dependent.
      c) Among adolescents who abuse substances, there is a higher incidence of mental health problems than in nonabusers.
         (1) Depression
         (2) Feelings of inferiority
         (3) Poor impulse control
         (4) Poor anger control

2. Women
   a) The incidence of alcoholism among women is increasing.
   b) Women react to alcohol differently than men do.
      (1) Women develop higher blood alcohol levels than men do when given the same amount of alcohol, adjusted for body weight.
      (2) Women taking oral contraceptives become more intoxicated and stay intoxicated longer than men do when drinking the same amount.
3. Psychiatric clients: Substance abuse reduces the efficacy of treatment.
4. Elderly clients
   a) Elderly clients often take multiple prescription medications.
   b) This can result in drug interaction and drug dependence problems.
   c) Drug interactions and substance abuse can cause symptoms of confusion that are misdiagnosed as dementia.
5. Nurses (see section I,F of this chapter)
6. Adult children of substance abusers (see section I,B,4 of this chapter)

D. Codependency
   1. Definition: A codependent person spends excessive amounts of time and energy taking care of a substance-abusing significant other at the expense of personal needs and desires.
   2. Characteristic behaviors
      a) Obtains self-esteem from being able to successfully control the behavior of himself/herself and others despite adverse consequences
      b) Assumes responsibility for meeting others' needs at the expense of personal needs
      c) Experiences anxiety and boundary distortions in situations of intimacy and separation
      d) Becomes involved in a relationship with another codependent person or with a person who has a personality disorder, a substance dependency, or an impulse disorder
      e) May demonstrate excessive denial, substance abuse, constricted emotions, stress-related medical illnesses, depression, compulsions, anxiety, and/or hypervigilance

E. Multiple drug abuse
   1. Synergistic effects of taking multiple drugs
      a) When taken together, some drugs result in a much more intense effect than would be the sum of the effect of each drug added together.
      b) The synergistic effects of certain substances can result in unintentional death.
   2. Antagonistic effects of drugs
      a) Some people who abuse substances take 1 drug to counteract another drug or to avoid withdrawal symptoms (e.g., cocaine and diazepam [Valium]); this type of substance abuse can lead to cross-addictions.

        b) Certain medications (e.g., naloxone hydrochloride [Narcan], an opiate antagonist) are given by health care workers to people who have overdosed to counteract the effects of the drug.

F. Nurses and substance abuse
  1. Substance abuse among nurses is a major problem.
    a) Among nurses, there is a much higher incidence of narcotic addiction (30%–50% higher) than among the general population.
    b) Nurses work under a great deal of stress and have easy access to drugs.
  2. A nurse has an ethical and legal responsibility to immediately report a colleague whom he/she suspects of abusing drugs.
    a) The life and career of the substance-abusing nurse are at risk.
    b) The lives and health of clients are at risk when the nurse is impaired because of substance abuse.

See text pages
_____

II. Types of substances commonly abused

A. Alcohol (DSM-IV)
  1. Maladaptive behavioral and psychologic changes associated with recent use and intoxication
    a) Inappropriate sexual behavior
    b) Aggressiveness
    c) Mood swings
    d) Impaired judgment
    e) Impaired social functioning
    f) Impaired occupational functioning
  2. Physical signs and symptoms of intoxication: at least 1 of the following
    a) Speech difficulties
    b) Incoordination
    c) Difficulty walking
    d) Attention deficits
    e) Memory deficits
    f) Nystagmus
    g) Stupor or coma
  3. Signs and symptoms of withdrawal: at least 2 of the following
    a) Autonomic hyperactivity (e.g., sweating, increased pulse rate)
    b) Hand tremor
    c) Difficulty sleeping
    d) Nausea or vomiting
    e) Hallucinations (visual, tactile, or auditory)
    f) Psychomotor agitation
    g) Anxiety
    h) Grand mal seizures

4. Alcohol and suicide
   a) Among people who abuse alcohol, there is a much higher incidence of attempted suicide than among the general population.
   b) Nurses must be alert to possible suicidal thoughts or behaviors among these clients.

B. Amphetamines (DSM-IV)
   1. Maladaptive behavioral and psychologic changes associated with recent use and intoxication
      a) Euphoria or flattened affect
      b) Changes in sociability
      c) Hyperalertness
      d) Interpersonal sensitivity
      e) Anxiety, tension, or anger
      f) Stereotyped compulsive behaviors (e.g., twitches, tics)
      g) Impaired judgment
   2. Physical signs and symptoms of intoxication: at least 2 of the following
      a) Increased or decreased heart rate
      b) Dilated pupils
      c) Hypertension or hypotension
      d) Sweating or chills
      e) Nausea or vomiting

Street Names of Psychoactive Substances

Amphetamines	Cannabis	Cocaine	Hallucinogens	Opioids	Phencyclidine
Bennies	Acapulco gold	Bernice	Acid	Boy	Angel dust
Black beauties	Bhang	Big bloke	Barrels	Cube juice	Boat
Brain pills	Bo bo bush	Big C	Big D	Dollies	Hog
Browns	Bush	C	Black magic	Doojee	Love boat
Cartwheels	Fu	Carrie	Blue heaven	Dujie	PCP
Confidence	Gage	Cecil	Brown dots	Foolish powder	Peace pill
drug	Grass	Cholley	Buttons	H	
Copilots	Griefo	Coke	California	Hairy	**Antianxiety**
Crank	Hay	Corrine	sunshine	Harry	**agents,**
Crinic	Hemp	Crystal	Domes	Hocus	**sedatives,**
Dexies	Indian hay	Dream	Flats	Hop	**hypnotics**
Diet pills	Jay	Dust	Green domes	Horse	Barbs
Eye openers	Keif	Flake	Hawaiian	Miss Emma	Cibas
Footballs	Loco weed	Girl	sunshine	Noise	Cibees
Hearts	Mary Jane	Gold dust	LSD	Pee	Downers
LA turnabouts	Mezz	Happy dust	Magic	Scag	Goofballs
Lid proppers	MJ	Heaven dust	mushroom	Schmack	Gorilla pills
Monster	Mootos	Nose candy	Mese	Smack	Meth
Peaches	Muggles	Schmack	Mind benders	Speedball	Peanuts
Pep pills	Mutah	Smack	Owsley's acid	(heroin plus	Sleeping pills
Roses	Pot	Snow	Peace tablet	cocaine)	Stoppers
Speed	Reefer	Speedball	Purple haze	TNT	Yellow jackets
Splivins	Rope	(cocaine plus	Squirrels	Unkie	
Spots	Smoke	heroin)	Strawberry field	White junk	
Superman pills	Splim	Star dust	Sunshine		
Truck drivers	Tea		White lightening		
Uppers	Weed		Window glass		

Figure 9–1
Street Names of Psychoactive Substances

       f) Weight loss

       g) Psychomotor agitation or depression

       h) Respiratory depression, chest pain, cardiac arrhythmias, or muscular weakness

       i) Dyskinesias, dystonias, confusion, seizures, or coma

   3. Signs and symptoms of withdrawal: dysphoria plus at least 2 of the following

       a) Fatigue

       b) Vivid nightmares

       c) Insomnia or hypersomnia

       d) Increased appetite

       e) Psychomotor agitation or suppression

C. Cannabis (DSM-IV)

   1. Maladaptive behavioral and psychologic changes associated with recent use and intoxication

       a) Euphoria

       b) Sense of time moving more slowly

       c) Impaired motor coordination

       d) Impaired judgment

       e) Social withdrawal

       f) Anxiety

   2. Physical signs and symptoms of intoxication: at least 2 of the following

       a) Red eyes

       b) Increased appetite

       c) Dry mouth

       d) Increased heart rate

   3. Signs and symptoms of withdrawal: Physical withdrawal does not occur with cannabis.

D. Cocaine (DSM-IV)

   1. Maladaptive behavioral and psychologic changes associated with recent use and intoxication

       a) Euphoria or flattened affect

       b) Changes in sociability

       c) Hyperalertness

       d) Interpersonal sensitivity

       e) Anxiety, tension, or anger

       f) Stereotyped compulsive behaviors

   2. Physical signs and symptoms of intoxication: at least 2 of the following

       a) Increased or decreased heart rate

       b) Dilated pupils

       c) Hypertension or hypotension

       d) Sweating or chills

e) Nausea or vomiting

f) Weight loss

g) Psychomotor agitation or suppression

h) Respiratory depression, chest pain, cardiac arrhythmias, or muscular weakness

i) Dyskinesias, dystonias, confusion, seizures, or coma

3. Signs and symptoms of withdrawal: dysphoria plus at least 2 of the following

a) Fatigue

b) Vivid nightmares

c) Insomnia or hypersomnia

d) Increased appetite

e) Psychomotor agitation or suppression

E. Hallucinogens (DSM-IV)

1. Maladaptive behavioral and psychologic changes associated with recent use and intoxication

a) Anxiety

b) Depression

c) Ideas of reference

d) Fear of going insane

e) Paranoia

f) Impaired judgment

g) Impaired social or occupational functioning

2. Perceptual changes associated with intoxication

a) Intensification of perceptions

b) Depersonalization

c) Derealization

d) Illusions

e) Hallucinations

f) Synesthesias

3. Physical signs and symptoms of intoxication: at least 2 of the following

a) Dilated pupils

b) Increased heart rate

c) Sweating

d) Heart palpitations

e) Blurred vision

f) Tremors

g) Incoordination

4. Flashbacks: perceptual changes that are reexperienced without taking additional hallucinogens

5. Signs and symptoms of withdrawal: Physical withdrawal does not occur with hallucinogens.

F. Opioids (DSM-IV)

1. Maladaptive behavioral and psychologic changes associated with recent use and intoxication

a) Initial euphoria

b) Indifference

c) Dysphoria

d) Psychomotor agitation or suppression

e) Impaired judgment

2. Physical signs and symptoms of intoxication: dilated or constricted pupils plus at least 1 of the following

a) Drowsiness or coma

b) Slurred speech

c) Memory or attention deficits

3. Signs and symptoms of withdrawal: at least 3 of the following

a) Dysphoria

b) Nausea or vomiting

c) Muscle pain

d) Watery eyes or runny nose

e) Dilated pupils, bristling hairs, or sweating

f) Diarrhea

g) Yawning

h) Fever

i) Insomnia

G. Phencyclidine (PCP) (DSM-IV)

1. Maladaptive behavioral and psychologic changes associated with recent use and intoxication

a) Belligerence

b) Physical aggressiveness

c) Impulsiveness

d) Unpredictability

e) Psychomotor agitation

f) Impaired judgment

2. Physical signs and symptoms of intoxication: at least 2 of the following

a) Nystagmus (horizontal or vertical)

b) Hypertension or increased heart rate

c) Elevated pain threshold or numbness

d) Dysarthria

e) Muscle rigidity

f) Seizures or coma

g) Abnormally acute hearing

3. Signs and symptoms of withdrawal: Physical withdrawal does not occur with phencyclidine.

H. Antianxiety agents, sedatives, and hypnotics

1. Maladaptive behavioral and psychologic changes associated with recent use and intoxication

a) Inappropriate sexual behavior

b) Aggressiveness

     c) Mood swings

     d) Impaired judgment

  2. Physical signs and symptoms of intoxication: at least 1 of the following

     a) Slurred speech

     b) Incoordination

     c) Difficulty walking

     d) Nystagmus

     e) Attention or memory deficits

     f) Stupor or coma

  3. Signs and symptoms of withdrawal: at least 2 of the following

     a) Autonomic hyperactivity

     b) Hand tremor

     c) Insomnia

     d) Nausea or vomiting

     e) Hallucinations or illusions (tactile, visual, or auditory)

     f) Psychomotor agitation

     g) Anxiety

     h) Grand mal seizures

III. Treatments

A. Substance abuse treatment centers

  1. Hospitalization: Some hospitals have specialized departments and personnel who can provide necessary care to detoxify and stabilize clients with acute symptoms of substance abuse.

  2. Residential treatment centers

     a) Long-term stays are usually necessary to successfully change a lifestyle that is centered on substance abuse.

     b) A healthier lifestyle, abstinence, and improved coping and social skills are among the treatment goals.

  3. Outpatient care

     a) Long-term stays in treatment centers are not feasible in all cases.

     b) Outpatient drug treatment programs allow the client to remain at home and to continue working while receiving treatment.

     c) This type of program is more effective for some types of substance abuse (e.g., multiple drug abuse) than for other types of abuse (e.g., heroin dependence).

  4. Employee assistance programs: offer counseling, information, and referrals in the workplace

B. Psychotherapy

  1. Individual therapy

  2. Group therapy

  3. Family therapy

C. 12-step programs

  1. These programs are based on the Twelve Steps of Alcoholics Anonymous (AA).

  2. Open meetings are held to help people who abuse substances as well as their children, spouses, and close friends (see Client Teaching Checklist, "12-Step Programs").

> See text pages
> _____

3. Unlike some self-help groups (e.g., Women for Sobriety), these programs include a religious component.

D. Drug therapies
   1. Disulfiram (Antabuse) interacts with all alcohol-based substances, causing serious physical symptoms and thus inhibiting alcohol use (see Client Teaching Checklists, "Substances to Avoid while Taking Disulfiram" and "Alcohol-Disulfiram Reaction").
   2. Clonidine hydrochloride (Catapres) blocks physical symptoms of opiate withdrawal and has been used investigationally for opiate detoxification.
   3. Naloxone hydrochloride (Narcan) is a narcotic antagonist and is used to treat opiate overdose.
   4. Methadone hydrochloride has the following uses.
      a) It is used to treat clients addicted to heroin: the uncontrolled and dangerous use of heroin is supplanted by the controlled use of oral methadone
      b) It can be used at maintenance levels (i.e., doses just large enough to prevent withdrawal symptoms without causing euphoria or intoxication).
      c) It can be used in gradually lower doses to aid detoxification.
   5. Bromocriptine mesylate (Parlodel) helps reduce craving for cocaine and is used during cocaine detoxification.

Twelve Steps of Alcoholics Anonymous

1. We admitted we were powerless over alcohol—that our lives had become unmanageable.
2. Came to believe that a Power greater than ourselves could restore us to sanity.
3. Made a decision to turn our will and our lives over to the care of God, as we understood Him.
4. Made a searching and fearless moral inventory of ourselves.
5. Admitted to God, to ourselves, and to another human being the exact nature of our wrongs.
6. Were entirely ready to have God remove all these defects of character.
7. Humbly asked Him to remove our shortcomings.
8. Made a list of all persons we had harmed, and became willing to make amends to them all.
9. Made direct amends to such people wherever possible, except when to do so would injure them or others.
10. Continued to take personal inventory and when we were wrong promptly admitted it.
11. Sought through prayer and meditation to improve our conscious contact with God, as we understood Him, praying only for knowledge of His will for us and the power to carry that out.
12. Having had a spiritual awakening as the result of these steps, we tried to carry this message to alcoholics, and to practice these principles in all our affairs.

SOURCE: The Twelve Steps are reprinted with permission of Alcoholics Anonymous World Services, Inc. Permission to reprint this material does not mean that AA has reviewed or approved the contents of this publication, nor that AA agrees with the views expressed herein. AA is a program of recovery from alcoholism *only*—use of the Twelve Steps in connection with programs and activities which are patterned after AA, but which address other problems, does not imply otherwise.

Figure 9–2
Twelve Steps of Alcoholics Anonymous

12-Step Programs

Inform clients who are substance abusers of the following programs:

✔ Alcoholics Anonymous (AA)
✔ Narcotics Anonymous (NA)

Inform relatives and friends of the client who is a substance abuser of the following programs:

✔ Al-Anon
✔ Alateen
✔ Adult Children of Alcoholics (ACOA)

IV. Essential nursing care

See text pages

A. Nursing assessment
1. Evaluate physical signs and symptoms.
   a) Consider unreported substance abuse in clients with unexplained or numerous minor injuries, needle marks, or inflammation or destruction of nasal septum.
   b) Check for drug-specific signs of intoxication, overdose, or withdrawal.
2. Obtain social history.
   a) Changes in job performance
   b) Changes in social relationships
   c) Changes in family relationships
   d) Other substance abuse within the family
3. Tailor assessments to client's level of functioning.
   a) Keep questions direct and brief (e.g., "What did you take?" and "How much did you take?").
   b) Obtain information from friends and family members if client is incoherent.
4. Take drug history.
   a) What drugs are used?
   b) How much and how often are they used?
   c) When did the client last use drugs?
   d) What are the client's prior experiences with withdrawal?
5. Obtain key information about the substance used by a client with a suspected overdose.
   a) What drugs were taken?
   b) How much was taken?
   c) When were they taken?
   d) What other drugs (and amounts) were taken in the past 24 hours and in the past week?
6. Be aware that people who abuse substances may deny or minimize the use patterns and negative consequences.
7. Do not challenge denials during assessment; confronting denial takes place during therapy.
8. Remain nonjudgmental even if client is uncooperative.

B. Nursing diagnoses
  1. Main NANDA nursing diagnoses
     a) Sensory/perceptual alterations
     b) Altered thought processes
     c) Anxiety
     d) Ineffective denial
  2. Additional NANDA nursing diagnoses
     a) Ineffective family coping
     b) Ineffective individual coping
     c) Altered family processes
     d) Altered health maintenance
     e) Hopelessness
     f) High risk for injury
     g) Altered nutrition
     h) Altered parenting
     i) Posttrauma response
     j) Altered role performance
     k) Self-esteem disturbance
     l) High risk for violence, self-directed
  3. Selected complete nursing diagnoses
     a) Altered thought processes related to history of cocaine abuse evidenced by client's statement that "the mind police are after me"
     b) Altered thought processes related to alcohol abuse evidenced by family reports of violent behavior and blackouts
     c) Pain related to narcotic withdrawal evidenced by client's verbal expressions and physical responses (holds stomach and rocks back and forth)
C. Planning (goal setting)
  1. General goals
     a) Maintain abstinence from psychoactive substances.
     b) Substitute healthy coping responses for substance abuse.

✔ CLIENT TEACHING CHECKLIST ✔

Substances to Avoid while Taking Disulfiram

Inform the client taking disulfiram (Antabuse) of the risk of toxic reaction associated with the following alcohol-based substances:

✔ Cough syrups
✔ Cold medicines
✔ Mouthwashes
✔ Food sauces made with wine
✔ Flavor extracts such as vanilla

✔ Vinegar
✔ After-shave lotions
✔ Skin products
✔ Rubbing compounds

Alcohol-Disulfiram Reaction

Teach the client taking disulfiram (Antabuse) about the following potential effects of drinking alcohol while using disulfiram:

✔ Facial flushing
✔ Increased heart rate
✔ Hypotension
✔ Severe headache
✔ Dizziness
✔ Confusion
✔ Nausea

✔ Vomiting
✔ Respiratory distress
✔ Chest pain
✔ Unconsciousness
✔ Convulsions
✔ Death

     c) Maintain safety, and promote physical comfort.

     d) Support client's efforts to modify addictive behavior.

     e) Identify and enlist social support systems for the client.

  2. Examples of specific goals

     a) Client will remain abstinent from psychoactive substances.

     b) Client will be able to identify 3 negative consequences in his/her life resulting from substance abuse.

     c) Client will attend at least 4 self-help meetings in the first week after discharge.

D. Nursing implementation (intervention)

  1. Provide substance-specific interventions during acute intoxication phase.

     a) If alcohol intoxication is suspected, allow effects of alcohol to subside before discussing possible goals with the client.

     b) If amphetamine (e.g., dextroamphetamine, methamphetamine) intoxication is suspected:

       (1) Administer ammonium chloride as ordered to acidify urine and promote excretion of the drug.

       (2) Administer phenothiazines as ordered to counteract psychotic reactions.

       (3) Monitor for hyperpyrexia, convulsions, respiratory distress, and cardiovascular shock.

     c) Cannabis (e.g., marijuana, hashish) intoxication: Nurses rarely encounter clients in need of treatment for cannabis intoxication.

     d) If cocaine intoxication is suspected:

       (1) Administer diazepam (Valium) as ordered to treat convulsions.

       (2) Monitor for hyperpyrexia, respiratory depression, and cardiac arrest.

     e) If hallucinogen (e.g., LSD, psilocybin, mescaline) intoxication is suspected:

       (1) Minimize external stimuli (keep lights, activity level, and noise level in room low).

       (2) Provide calm reassurance to "talk down" the client.

MAST Responses of Hospitalized Alcoholics and Nonalcoholic Controls (in Percents)

Points	Questions	Alcoholics (N = 116)		Nonalcoholics (N = 103)	
		Yes	No	Yes	No
2	*1. Do you feel you are a normal drinker?	14	86	99	1
2	2. Have you ever awakened the morning after some drinking the night before and found that you could not remember a part of the evening before?	80	20	18	82
1	3. Does your wife (or parents) ever worry or complain about your drinking?	86	12**	7	93
2	*4. Can you stop drinking without a struggle after one or two drinks?	34	66	98	2
1	5. Do you ever feel bad about your drinking?	91	9	6	94
2	*6. Do friends or relatives think you are a normal drinker?	15	82***	99	1
0	7. Do you ever try to limit your drinking to certain times of the day or to certain places?	53	47	11	89
2	*8. Are you always able to stop drinking when you want to?	36	64	96	4
5	9. Have you ever attended a meeting of Alcoholics Anonymous (AA)?	65	35	0	100
1	10. Have you gotten into fights when drinking?	30	70	9	91
2	11. Has drinking ever created problems with you and your wife?	66	22†	7	86†
2	12. Has your wife (or other family member) ever gone to anyone for help about your drinking?	37	63	0	100
2	13. Have you ever lost friends or girlfriends/boyfriends because of drinking?	46	54	1	99
2	14. Have you ever gotten into trouble at work because of drinking?	52	48	0	100
2	15. Have you ever lost a job because of drinking?	39	61	0	100
2	16. Have you ever neglected your obligations, your family, or your work for two or more days in a row because you were drinking?	61	39	0	100
1	17. Do you ever drink before noon?	85	15	22	78
2	18. Have you ever been told you have liver trouble? Cirrhosis?	31	69	1	99
2	19. Have you ever had delirium tremens (DTs), severe shaking, heard voices or seen things that weren't there after heavy drinking?	49	51	0	100
5	20. Have you ever gone to anyone for help about your drinking?	28	72	0	100
5	21. Have you ever been in a hospital because of drinking?	45	55	1	99
2	22. Have you ever been a patient in a psychiatric hospital or on a psychiatric ward of a general hospital where drinking was part of the problem?	21	79	0	100
2	23. Have you ever been seen at a psychiatric or mental health clinic, or gone to a doctor, social worker, or clergyman for help with an emotional problem in which drinking had played a part?	31	69	0	100
2	24. Have you ever been arrested, even for a few hours, because of drunk behavior?	49	51	4	96
2	25. Have you ever been arrested for drunk driving or driving after drinking?	45	55	1	99

* Negative responses are alcoholic responses.
** Two (2 percent) were single, with both parents out of the picture.
*** Three (3 percent) gave no response to this question.
† Fourteen (12 percent) of the alcoholics and seven (7 percent) of the control group were single.

SOURCE: Reprinted from *American Journal of Psychiatry*, vol. 127, pp. 1653–1658, 1971. With permission from the American Psychiatric Association.

Figure 9–3
Michigan Alcoholism Screening Test (MAST): An Assessment Tool

(3) Take steps to ensure safety of the client and caregivers.
  (a) Apply restraints as ordered.
  (b) Provide continuous observation and monitoring.
(4) Initiate gastric lavage as ordered.
f) If opioid (e.g., heroin, morphine, meperidine [Demerol]) intoxication is suspected:
  (1) Administer naloxone hydrochloride (Narcan) as ordered to counteract central nervous system effects of substance.
  (2) Monitor for respiratory depression, coma, shock, and convulsions.
g) If phencyclidine (PCP) intoxication is suspected:
  (1) Do not engage client in interaction; a violent reaction may result.
  (2) Administer cranberry juice or ascorbic acid as ordered to promote excretion of the drug.
h) If antianxiety agent, sedative, or hypnotic (e.g., barbiturates, benzodiazepines [diazepam], methaqualone) intoxication is suspected:
  (1) In client who is conscious:
    (a) Maintain conscious state.
    (b) Administer activated charcoal as ordered to promote absorption of drug.
    (c) Induce vomiting as ordered.
    (d) Monitor vital signs.
  (2) In client who is unconscious:
    (a) Maintain clear airway.
    (b) Initiate intravenous fluids as ordered.
    (c) Initiate gastric lavage as ordered.
    (d) Monitor vital signs.

 SKIDMORE PSYCHIATRIC HOSPITAL

BEHAVIORAL CONTRACT

I hereby agree to:

Attend AA meetings at least 5 times a week.
Attend all scheduled individual and group therapy sessions.
Take Antabuse as prescribed.
Call my counselor if I feel the urge to drink.

Client signature	Date
Nurse signature	Date

Figure 9–4
Behavioral Contract

2. Assist in the development of adequate coping mechanisms.
    a) Help client admit to substance abuse problem.
    b) Advise client to attend meetings of self-help group regularly.
    c) Have client identify situations that trigger urge to use substance.
    d) Develop written contract with client stipulating behavior changes.
    e) Have client substitute healthy compulsion (e.g., exercise) for unhealthy one.
3. In cases of overdose, do the following.
    a) Assess circumstances of overdose to determine whether it was accidental or intentional.
    b) Assess for risk of suicide.
4. Provide interventions during detoxification.
    a) Ask client about other drug use to identify multiple drug use, which may complicate detoxification and treatment.
    b) Anticipate the possibility of seizures, and ensure that emergency equipment is available.
    c) Observe for signs of secret drug use or hoarding of drugs; notify physician if drug use is suspected.
    d) Collect blood and urine specimens as ordered to ensure compliance.
5. Provide interventions during early recovery/inpatient treatment.
    a) Assist client in overcoming denial by sharing objective evidence of his/her substance abuse (e.g., "You've had a lot of auto accidents. Had you been drinking before they happened?").
    b) Maintain nonjudgmental, accepting attitude.
    c) Express confidence in the client's ability to overcome substance abuse.
    d) Establish firm rules regarding behavioral expectations (e.g., remaining abstinent, attending meetings, making his/her bed in the morning).
    e) Provide client education about recovery process (see Client Teaching Checklist, "The Recovery Process").

✔ CLIENT TEACHING CHECKLIST ✔

The Recovery Process

Explanations to the client:

✔ Normal physical and psychologic changes occur during the first several months of abstinence.
    — Weight gain
    — Heightened experience of feelings such as sadness
✔ You must develop new patterns of behavior with your family and peer groups.
✔ You may need to develop new peer groups.

6. Provide interventions during aftercare and ongoing recovery.
   a) Counsel clients about the risk of fetal damage resulting from alcohol or drug abuse; emphasize that damage can occur if either parent abuses drugs.
   b) Make referrals to community support systems, and provide follow-up.

E. Nursing evaluation
   1. Assess the client's progress.
      a) Client begins to take responsibility for his/her actions.
      b) Client confronts his/her problems honestly, without resorting to denial or rationalization.
      c) Client improves his/her problem-solving skills.
      d) Client is less compulsive and impulsive.
      e) Client is able to set goals and work toward them.
      f) Client can communicate in a nondefensive way.
      g) Client reacts appropriately to daily stress and is able to manage stress without the use of psychoactive substances.
      h) Client participates in healthy social and recreational activities.
      i) Client has a solid social support network.
      j) Client is productive at work.
      k) Client is able to maintain meaningful and healthy interpersonal relationships.
      l) Dysfunctional family patterns have been addressed and altered.
      m) Healthy patterns have been established for family conflict resolution and expression of feelings.
      n) Client is aware of additional community resources and is willing to use them.
   2. Establish and review postdischarge goals with the family.
   3. Assess one's own concerns and anxieties (see Nurse Alert, "Exploring Personal Feelings about Substance Abuse").
   4. Revise goals and care plan as necessary.

! NURSE *ALERT* !

Exploring Personal Feelings about Substance Abuse

- Acknowledge to peers and superiors feelings of anger and frustration regarding clients who relapse or engage in manipulative or deceptive behavior.
- Identify attitudes you may have that enable a client's substance abuse.
  —Acceptance of client's denial
  —Sympathy for client's reasons for abuse
  —Belief that substance abuse problem is not physical but moral
- Seek feedback from and consult with peers and superiors.

1. Anthony has been admitted to an alcoholism treatment center. During history taking, which of the following assessment findings represents a common risk factor for alcoholism?

   a. Anthony experienced blackouts during his first few drinking experiences.
   b. Anthony was always able to drink more than his peers before showing signs of intoxication.
   c. In Anthony's first drinking experiences, 1–2 drinks produced signs of intoxication.
   d. Alcohol was a part of family rituals and celebrations during Anthony's childhood.

2. The nurse should suspect codependency in a client who:

   a. Leaves his/her own needs unmet while striving to meet others' needs.
   b. Expresses helplessness and inability to control his/her own behavior.
   c. Demonstrates difficulty forming intimate relationships.
   d. Behaves in disorganized or unpredictable ways.

3. Mr. Lundgren, who has a history of alcohol abuse, has been admitted to the hospital for detoxification. During the first 2–3 days after admission, the nurse should anticipate that Mr. Lundgren will demonstrate:

   a. Ataxic gait.
   b. Psychomotor retardation.
   c. Bradycardia.
   d. Insomnia.

4. During the first weeks of abstinence, the client with alcoholism should be encouraged to eat a diet high in:

   a. B vitamins.
   b. Calcium.
   c. Vitamin D.
   d. Fiber.

5. The parents of 14-year-old Meg Reynard are concerned that she may be abusing marijuana (cannabis). As the nurse explains the signs of marijuana intoxication to the Reynards, which of the following should be included?

   a. Red eyes
   b. Anorexia
   c. Excessive salivation
   d. Social intrusiveness

6. Andy Baines, age 30, is brought to the hospital emergency department by 2 friends who report that Andy developed chest pains at a party. He is diaphoretic and agitated. His vital signs are: temperature 99°F, pulse 112, respirations 14, blood pressure 164/86. Based on these assessments, the nurse should suspect intoxication with:

   a. Narcotics.
   b. Cannabis.
   c. Hallucinogens.
   d. Cocaine.

7. Helene Figueroa is experiencing symptoms of alcohol withdrawal during her hospitalization for minor surgery. She reports that she never drinks more than a glass of wine with dinner and attributes her symptoms to surgical complications. She refuses to talk further with the nurse. The most appropriate nursing diagnosis for Ms. Figueroa at this time is:

   a. Self-esteem disturbance.
   b. Ineffective denial.
   c. Self-care deficit.
   d. Social isolation.

8. When a client is admitted to the hospital for medical management of opiate withdrawal, the nurse should anticipate administering:

   a. Naloxone hydrochloride (Narcan).
   b. Clonidine hydrochloride (Catapres).
   c. Disulfiram (Antabuse).
   d. Bromocriptine mesylate (Parlodel).

9. Nineteen-year-old Tommy is brought to the hospital emergency department by his parents, who report that he has a history of using angel dust (phencyclidine [PCP]). They found him sitting and staring into space. He did not respond when his name was called. When the nurse approaches to take his blood pressure, Tommy raises his fists and yells, "Get away from me!" Which of the following interventions is indicated at this point in Tommy's care?

   a. He should be placed in soft restraints.
   b. Physical care should be deferred until he is less agitated.
   c. One staff member should be assigned to remain with Tommy at all times.
   d. He should be placed in a seclusion room.

10. The client who is being treated with disulfiram (Antabuse) should be cautioned to avoid:

    a. Aged cheeses.
    b. Decongestant nasal sprays.
    c. Over-the-counter analgesics.
    d. After-shave lotion.

11. David, age 16, has begun attending Narcotics Anonymous (NA) meetings while undergoing inpatient treatment for opiate addiction. His parents are questioning why David should continue going to NA meetings after discharge. Which of the following statements by the nurse best explains the benefits of NA?

    a. Trained group leaders help addicts examine the reasons for their drug use.
    b. NA provides an educational program to make clients aware of the consequences of their drug use.
    c. Meetings allow the client to form peer relationships that support abstinence.
    d. NA provides weekly urine testing for early detection of drug use.

12. Diazepam (Valium) was prescribed for Arlette, who is suffering severe anxiety over a recent divorce. She is brought to the hospital emergency department by her mother, who found her mumbling incoherently. The empty Valium bottle was on the floor beside her. The nurse should:

    a. Initiate seizure precautions.
    b. Encourage her to drink cranberry juice.
    c. Administer naloxone hydrochloride (Narcan) as ordered.
    d. Initiate cardiac monitoring.

ANSWERS

1. **Correct answer is b.** Studies have shown that people who abuse alcohol metabolize ethanol more rapidly than nonabusers, which produces a higher tolerance for alcohol. This is apparent even early in the client's drinking history.

   a. Although blackouts can occur at any point in the progression of the disease, they become more likely as the alcoholism becomes more severe. They are not common in the early stages.
   c. Becoming intoxicated after 1–2 drinks indicates a low tolerance for alcohol, which is not a common feature in the history of alcoholics.
   d. The presence of alcohol at family gatherings is not, by itself, a risk factor. A pattern of abuse in the family may be a risk factor, but modeling of appropriate use may actually decrease the risk of future abuse.

2. **Correct answer is a.** The codependent person tends to assume responsibility for meeting others' needs at the expense of his/her own needs.

   b. The codependent person derives self-esteem from the ability to control his/her own and others' behavior.
   c. The codependent person does form intimate relationships and may experience distortion of boundaries in such relationships.
   d. The codependent person is more likely to be compulsive or rigid in his/her behavior patterns than to be unpredictable.

3. **Correct answer is d.** Sleep disturbances are common during alcohol withdrawal.

   a. Ataxic gait, or difficulty walking, is associated with alcohol intoxication, not withdrawal.
   b. Alcohol withdrawal produces psychomotor agitation, not retardation.
   c. Autonomic hyperactivity occurs with alcohol withdrawal and is manifested by sweating, tachycardia, and high blood pressure.

4. **Correct answer is a.** Alcohol causes malabsorption of B vitamins. Supplementing B vitamins improves metabolism of other foods and may reduce the peripheral neuropathies often seen in alcoholics.

   b. Calcium is not altered by alcohol. Alcohol increases urinary excretion of potassium and magnesium, which may need to be supplemented.
   c. Vitamin D is not directly affected by alcohol use.
   d. Increased fiber in the early recovery period may worsen diarrhea. Fiber intake should be increased gradually.

5. **Correct answer is a.** Marijuana causes dilation of the capillaries in the eyes, producing a characteristic reddening of the sclerae.

   b. Increased appetite ("the munchies") is characteristic of marijuana use.
   c. Marijuana intoxication produces dry mouth.
   d. Social withdrawal is more likely with marijuana use.

6. **Correct answer is d.** Cardiac problems with chest pain are most likely to occur with cocaine or amphetamine use. Hypertension, tachycardia, respiratory depression, and agitation are typical of stimulant drugs.

   a. Narcotics are depressants and would produce drowsiness, respiratory depression, hypotension, and bradycardia in the initial stages.
   b. Although tachycardia may occur with cannabis use, chest pain would be unlikely. The other physical signs reported are not common with cannabis use.

   c. Hallucinogens might produce the physical changes described but do not usually progress to chest pain. Paranoia or fear of insanity is likely to occur with hallucinogen use.

7. **Correct answer is b.** Denial is the most universal defense mechanism of substance abusers. Prolonged denial eventually becomes maladaptive, so ineffective denial is an appropriate diagnosis for the client who is experiencing physical problems as a result of alcohol abuse.

   a. Self-esteem disturbances are common in alcoholics. However, this interaction does not provide evidence to support this diagnosis.
   c. Self-care deficits are uncommon in alcoholics, except when they are severely intoxicated or in the very late stages of alcohol-induced dementia.
   d. Refusing to talk with the nurse who has presented evidence of the client's alcohol abuse is evidence of denial. There is no indication that she is isolated from others.

8. **Correct answer is b.** Clonidine hydrochloride has been found to suppress opioid withdrawal symptoms.

   a. Naloxone hydrochloride is an opiate antagonist, which is used to reverse effects of overdose. It would worsen withdrawal symptoms.
   c. Disulfiram is sometimes used to help alcoholics maintain abstinence. It has no effect on opiate withdrawal symptoms.
   d. Bromocriptine mesylate is sometimes used to reduce the craving for cocaine during detoxification. It has no effect on opiate withdrawal symptoms.

9. **Correct answer is b.** Every effort should be made to decrease stimulation. Any physical care that is not absolutely necessary should be deferred, since any violation of the client's personal space may escalate his agitation to violence.

   a. Restraints will most likely increase the client's agitation. Efforts to restrain him could lead to violence against staff.

c. No staff person should ever be alone with the client who is intoxicated with PCP. Whenever a member of the staff needs to approach, sufficient personnel should be present to restrain the client if necessary.

d. Clients intoxicated with PCP tend to become paranoid. The least restrictive environment possible should be used to avoid exacerbating the paranoia.

10. **Correct answer is d.** Clients using disulfiram must avoid products containing alcohol. Since significant amounts of alcohol can be absorbed through the skin, this includes topical products.

    a and **b.** Aged cheeses and decongestant nasal sprays should be avoided by clients using monoamine oxidase inhibitors (MAOIs). They do not affect clients taking disulfiram.

    c. Over-the-counter analgesics often contain aspirin. They increase the risk of bleeding in clients who are using large amounts of alcohol. They would not interact with disulfiram.

11. **Correct answer is c.** Peer support is especially effective for adolescents, who respond better to peers than to authority figures. It will be important for David to form peer relationships that support abstinence rather than drug use.

    a. NA is a self-help group. There are no trained leaders or counselors.

    b. NA is not an educational program. It is a self-help group based on the Twelve Steps developed by Alcoholics Anonymous (AA).

    d. NA is completely voluntary and does not mandate any type of monitoring for drug use.

12. **Correct answer is a.** Seizures are a potential complication of intoxication with CNS depressants. Seizure precautions should be in effect for the client until the drug has been cleared from her system.

    b. Drinking cranberry juice would speed excretion of amphetamines or PCP. It has no effect on duration of action of benzodiazepines.

    c. Naloxone hydrochloride is an opiate antagonist. It would have no effect in benzodiazepine overdose.

    d. Cardiac monitoring would be important after an overdose with tricyclic antidepressants, cocaine, or amphetamines. It is not indicated in benzodiazepine overdose.

10
Eating Disorders

NURSING HIGHLIGHTS

1. Eating disorders, which include anorexia nervosa, bulimia nervosa, and obesity, involve disruptions in normal eating behaviors.
2. Anorexia nervosa is often difficult to treat successfully and leads to death in a significant percentage of its victims.
3. Bulimia nervosa reflects poor impulse control and unrealistic expectations about weight.
4. Obesity caused by compulsive eating has many features in common with substance abuse and other addictive disorders.
5. Nurse must be aware of his/her own attitudes and body image concerns and must understand that eating disorders can be life-threatening.
6. The main goals of nursing care for a client with an eating disorder are to preserve life, to help the client develop healthful eating behaviors, and to help the client and family gain insight into the causes of the disorder.

GLOSSARY

body image—a person's perception of his/her physical appearance; important aspect of concept of self
cachexia—a state of physical wasting, emaciation, and weakness
chipmunk facies—facial characteristic of bulimia caused by enlarged parotid gland
lanugo—fine, downy hair that can appear on a person with anorexia nervosa; also covers a fetus during the second half of the gestation period

self-esteem—the degree of acceptance, respect, and approval accorded to oneself

tetany—physical condition characterized by muscle spasms, cramps, convulsions, and hyperflexion of the wrists and ankles

ENHANCED OUTLINE

I. General concepts

See text pages
_____

A. Anorexia nervosa (DSM-IV)
1. Refusal to maintain body weight at or above a minimally normal weight for age and height (body weight less than 85% of what is expected)
2. Intense fear in underweight person of gaining weight or becoming fat
3. Body image disturbance; undue influence of body weight or shape on self-evaluation or denial of seriousness of current low body weight
4. Amenorrhea in postmenarchal females for at least 3 consecutive menstrual cycles
5. May occur with or without bingeing or purging behaviors

B. Bulimia nervosa (DSM-IV)
1. Recurrent binge-eating behavior: eating in a discrete time period an amount of food that is more than most people would eat; a feeling of a lack of control over eating during the binge
2. Recurrent inappropriate compensatory behavior to prevent weight gain (e.g., self-induced vomiting; use of laxatives, diuretics, or other medication; fasting; excessive exercise)
3. Occurrence of both behaviors an average of at least twice a week for 3 months
4. Undue influence of body weight or shape on self-evaluation

C. Obesity due to compulsive eating (not specifically defined in DSM-IV)
1. Developmental obesity: begins in childhood; is believed to result from overfeeding and/or the attachment of high emotional value to food
2. Reactive obesity: occurs later in life as a maladaptive coping mechanism for stress

D. General symptoms
1. Anorexia nervosa
   a) Cachexia
   b) Lanugo
   c) Hair loss
   d) Yellowish skin
   e) Cyanosis of the extremities
   f) Amenorrhea
   g) Bradycardia
2. Bulimia nervosa
   a) Chipmunk facies
   b) Chronic hoarseness
   c) Tooth decay

        d) Electrolyte imbalances

        e) Dehydration

     3. Obesity due to compulsive eating

        a) Excessive weight

        b) Hypertension

        c) Heart disease

        d) Diabetes

E. Theories of causation

    1. General concepts

        a) Although each eating disorder is distinct, it is believed that certain issues are common to all of them.

           (1) Problems with the ability to identify and express needs

           (2) Inadequate coping mechanisms

           (3) Need for self-control

        b) Biologic causes of eating disorders are not widely accepted among researchers, but investigations continue.

        c) Approximately 95% of those with an eating disorder are female; onset usually occurs between ages 13 and 35.

    2. Causal models

        a) Psychodynamic model: Eating disorders have their roots in inadequate separation from the mother, development of self-critical behaviors, and perception of the body as "the enemy."

        b) Family model: Families of persons with anorexia share 5 characteristics, each of which promotes anorexic behavior.

           (1) Enmeshment: Family members have difficulty identifying and meeting their individual needs.

           (2) Overprotectiveness: The family—especially the parents—intervene in the client's decision-making process.

           (3) Rigidity: The family exhibits only a limited range of behaviors in response to a given situation; when a given behavior is not effective, family members may intensify the behavior rather than try something else.

           (4) Lack of conflict resolution: The family cannot solve problems.

           (5) Involvement of the child with an eating disorder in parental conflict: The child is used by 1 parent against the other.

        c) Sociocultural model

           (1) Eating disorders may arise from conflicts over changing roles of women and from the transmission of these conflicts from mother to daughter.

           (2) Anorexia and bulimia are seen as compulsions grounded in attempts to attain society's current ideal body shape.

           (3) Compulsive eating is seen as an unconscious rebellion against the ideal of slimness.

F. Treatments
   1. Drug therapies (play supportive role)
      a) Tranquilizers (e.g., phenothiazines)
      b) Antidepressants (e.g., fluoxetine hydrochloride, imipramine, chlorpromazine)
         (1) Depression often accompanies eating disorders.
         (2) Treatment of depression can aid in resolving the eating disorder.
      c) Appetite regulators (e.g., amphetamines)
         (1) Short-term effectiveness in obesity
         (2) High risk of developing dependence
      d) Anticonvulsants: Effectiveness has not been established.
   2. Psychotherapy
      a) Focuses on body image, identification and expression of needs, and control issues
      b) May include individual, group, or family therapy
   3. Inpatient treatment for anorexia nervosa
      a) Used for severe cases
         (1) Loss of more than 15% of body weight
         (2) Refusal to eat
         (3) Suicidal thoughts
         (4) Medical emergencies (e.g., cardiac arrhythmias)
      b) Provides nutritional rehabilitation
         (1) An individualized diet is planned for a steady weight gain of 2–3 lb per week.
         (2) Weight goal is typically established in low-normal range for height and body frame.
         (3) Hyperalimentation and tube feedings may be necessary if client fails to show sufficient weight gain.
         (4) Attempts are made to establish normal eating patterns, not simply to achieve weight gain.
      c) Provides behavior modification: These techniques are important during early treatment, when the physical and psychologic effects of starvation interfere with insight-oriented therapy.
      d) Provides psychotherapy to address underlying issues
   4. Inpatient treatment for bulimia
      a) Used in cases in which binge-purge cycle cannot be controlled with outpatient treatment or in which significant medical or psychiatric emergencies exist
      b) Focuses on establishing healthy eating behaviors
      c) Involves insight-oriented psychotherapy to help client develop effective coping mechanisms
      d) Addresses other manifestations of anxiety that emerge as eating behaviors change (e.g., panic attacks, phobias)
   5. Inpatient treatment for obesity
      a) Used for treatment of serious medical problems
      b) May involve surgical treatment for obesity (e.g., gastric stapling)
      c) Used when there is a need for rapid supervised weight loss

II. Essential nursing care

See text pages

_____

A. Nursing assessment
  1. Check for signs and symptoms of eating disorder.
  2. Make a thorough weight assessment.
     a) Present weight
     b) Recent gains and/or losses
     c) Body image
  3. Assess eating patterns.
     a) How much and how often the client eats
     b) Foods eaten
     c) Presence of binge-purge cycles or rituals
     d) Feelings about food and eating behaviors
     e) Impact of eating behaviors on the client's daily activities
     f) Level of impulse control in other areas (drug use, sexual promiscuity, lying, stealing)
  4. Assess activity levels for presence of compulsive exercise.
  5. Assess family.
     a) Functional and problem-solving abilities
     b) Problem areas, patterns, and issues
     c) Ability to express emotions
     d) Family history of eating disorders
     e) Parental marital conflict
     f) Responses to client's eating behavior and weight (e.g., denial, anger, ridicule)
     g) Family patterns of eating-related behavior

B. Nursing diagnoses
  1. Main NANDA nursing diagnoses
     a) Body image disturance
     b) Altered nutrition, less than body requirements (anorexia)
     c) Altered nutrition, more than body requirements (obesity)
     d) Potential for violence, self-directed
  2. Additional NANDA nursing diagnoses
     a) Anxiety
     b) Decreased cardiac output (related to electrolyte imbalances)
     c) Ineffective individual coping
     d) Ineffective family coping
     e) Altered family processes
     f) Potential fluid volume deficit
     g) Self-esteem disturbance
  3. Selected complete nursing diagnoses
     a) Altered nutrition, less than body requirements, related to fear of weight gain evidenced by loss of 35 lb in past 3 months

      b) Body image disturbance related to inability to realistically perceive body size evidenced by denial of extreme thinness

C. Planning (goal setting)
   1. General goals
      a) Prevent infliction of self-harm.
      b) Promote insight into underlying issues.
      c) Alter self-destructive eating patterns.
      d) Develop healthy coping mechanisms.
   2. Examples of specific goals
      a) Client will gain 1 kg per week.
      b) Frequency of purging will be reduced by 90% within 2 weeks of beginning treatment.
      c) Client will promote self-esteem by identifying 2 positive personality traits.

D. Nursing implementation (intervention)
   1. General interventions for eating disorders
      a) Educate client about healthy eating patterns, and focus on behavior rather than weight.
      b) Work to establish trust: Listen empathically to client; avoid judgments and confrontations, especially early in treatment.
      c) Begin to explore family issues with client and family.
      d) Administer medications as ordered, and observe for side effects.
      e) Regularly assess client for suicide potential.
      f) Assist client in development of healthy coping mechanisms.
      g) Promote social interaction to reduce feelings of isolation.
      h) Manage personal feelings and attitudes toward clients with eating disorders (see Nurse Alert, "Managing Personal Reactions to Clients with Eating Disorders").
   2. Specific interventions for anorexia nervosa
      a) Administer hyperalimentation and/or tube feedings, as ordered.
      b) Explore client's feelings during inpatient rehabilitation to assess potential for reverting to anorexic behaviors after discharge.
      c) Monitor temperature, respiration, blood pressure, and pulse daily.
      d) Observe for signs of tetany and muscle cramping to detect electrolyte imbalances and hypokalemia.

! NURSE *ALERT* !

Managing Personal Reactions to Clients with Eating Disorders
- Explore your personal feelings and attitudes toward clients with eating disorders.
  —Personal body image concerns can result in overidentification with client.
  —Feelings of despondency can be triggered by client's depression.
  —Feelings of anger can result if you fail to view eating disorder as being serious.
- Acknowledge your feelings to your peers and superiors.
- Seek feedback from and consult with peers and superiors.

        e) Observe and measure caloric intake and urinary and fecal output.

        f) Observe for evidence of rituals, especially those that may disguise reduced eating (e.g., moving food around, spilling food, spitting food into a napkin).

        g) Observe for signs of purging after meals.

        h) Observe activity level, especially for excessive exercise.

        i) Weigh at same time each day with client in light clothing.

        j) Establish contract with client to achieve minimal safe weight as a condition of discharge.

        k) Reassure client that rapid or excessive weight gain is not the goal of treatment.

        l) Permit increasing control over treatment plan as the client's eating behaviors become more normal.

        m) Assist client in establishing contacts with community support systems.

    3. Specific interventions for bulimia

        a) Observe for signs of purging after meals.

        b) Monitor temperature, respiration, blood pressure, and pulse daily.

        c) Observe for signs of tetany and muscle cramping to detect electrolyte imbalances and hypokalemia.

        d) Establish contract with client to stop or reduce frequency of bingeing and purging by a specific date.

    4. Specific interventions for compulsive eating

        a) Provide positive feedback to promote client's self-esteem.

        b) Review with the client his/her personal strengths and supports.

        c) Observe for signs of depression.

        d) Observe for signs of furtive eating.

        e) Weigh at same time each day with client in light clothing.

E. Nursing evaluation

    1. Review goals, and assess progress.

        a) Anorexic or obese client achieves weight goals or makes progress toward those goals.

        b) Bulimic client reduces or eliminates bingeing and purging behaviors.

        c) Client gains insight into his/her eating disorder.

        d) Client develops effective coping mechanisms.

        e) Client establishes healthy eating behaviors.

        f) Client is involved in aftercare (e.g., self-help groups, psychotherapy).

        g) Progress has been made on family issues.

        h) Medical problems (e.g., cardiac output, hypokalemia) are adequately controlled.

        i) Postdischarge goals have been established and have been reviewed with the family.

        j) Nurse addresses his/her own concerns and anxieties.

    2. Revise goals and care plan as necessary.

1. Kathy Richards, 15 years old, is 5′6″ and weighs 85 lb. For the past 6 months she has exercised vigorously and restricted her food intake. Prior to this 6-month period, she weighed 120 lb. She is admitted to an eating disorders unit of a general hospital. As the nurse collects assessment data, which finding would support the presence of anorexia nervosa?

   a. Low motivation
   b. Poor school performance
   c. Distorted body image
   d. Poor impulse control

2. During the first week of Kathy's treatment, the nurse identifies the nursing diagnosis of altered nutrition, less than body requirements, related to refusal to eat as evidenced by low body weight. The best nursing care goal related to this diagnosis is:

   a. Kathy will state how she feels about food.
   b. Kathy will gain 1–2 lb within 1 week.
   c. Kathy will improve her attitude toward food.
   d. Kathy will agree to eat 3 meals a day.

3. Each evening, Kathy's mother visits the unit and asks Kathy if she has eaten or had a bowel movement that day. Mrs. Richards states to the primary nurse, "If Kathy doesn't start eating soon, I'll just die." Which common characteristic of families of clients who have anorexia is demonstrated by this statement?

   a. Enmeshment
   b. Denial
   c. Rigidity
   d. Scapegoating

4. As a result of frequent purging, a client with a diagnosis of bulimia nervosa is most likely to develop which of the following conditions?

   a. Cachexia
   b. Amenorrhea
   c. Dehydration
   d. Hair loss

5. Early in treatment, which of the following nursing interventions would most effectively discourage purging by the client with a diagnosis of bulimia?

   a. Observe client for 1 hour after meals.
   b. Weigh client 3 times a day.
   c. Provide teaching about nutrition.
   d. Contract for immediate cessation of purging.

6. During a nursing assessment of a client with a diagnosis of bulimia, which of the following conditions would most likely indicate hypokalemia (low serum potassium)?

   a. Diarrhea
   b. Urinary retention
   c. Muscle spasms
   d. Hyperactivity

7. The most appropriate nursing care goal for Charles, a client with a diagnosis of bulimia, is:

   a. Charles will follow the diet he is given.
   b. Charles will avoid buying large quantities of food.
   c. Charles will identify situations that cause anxiety.
   d. Charles will develop strategies to help him control his impulse to eat.

8. After Charles misses his individual counseling session with his primary nurse, he admits that he went to the hospital cafeteria and ate "tons" of food and vomited in the woods behind the hospital. The best response by the nurse is:

   a. "If you miss your appointments, you are never going to get well."
   b. "I know you were probably upset about something today. Don't feel bad. Everybody gets upset sometimes."
   c. "Let's try to figure out exactly how much you ate today."
   d. "You must have been upset today. Let's try to figure out why."

9. Reactive obesity, which occurs in adulthood, is believed to be most closely associated with:

   a. Maladaptive coping.
   b. Overfeeding in childhood.
   c. Depression.
   d. A metabolic disorder.

ANSWERS

1. **Correct answer is c.** Despite muscle wasting and loss of at least 15% of body weight, clients who have anorexia deny their low body weight and frequently complain of being fat.

   a and **b.** Clients who have anorexia are frequently highly motivated academically and professionally.
   d. Clients who have anorexia exhibit extreme control of their impulses, as manifested by their ability to deny hunger.

2. **Correct answer is b.** Weight gain of 1–2 lb in 1 week is a realistic, measurable nursing goal. Rather than engaging the client in control issues related to food intake, the goal of weight gain is established.

   a. This nursing goal is not directly related to the nursing diagnosis. Also, clients who have anorexia frequently are not able to examine feelings related to food until later in treatment.
   c. This nursing goal is not directly related to the nursing diagnosis.
   d. This nursing goal is related to the diagnosis, but it is not a realistic goal for the first week of treatment.

3. **Correct answer is a.** Enmeshment is characterized by overinvolvement among family members and includes lack of appropriate boundaries between family members.

   b. Denial would be evidenced by a family member who refuses to acknowledge the seriousness of anorexia.
   c. Rigidity would be evidenced by the family's use of a narrow range of behaviors in dealing with problems or situations.

   d. Scapegoating would be evidenced by blaming the client as being the source of all the family's problems.

4. **Correct answer is c.** Use of laxatives, diuretics, and vomiting to purge leads to dehydration.

   a. Clients who have bulimia are usually of normal weight or slightly overweight. Cachexia, or physical wasting, is common in anorexia.
   b and **d.** Amenorrhea and hair loss are not consistent with the effects of bulimia. They are associated with anorexia.
   d. Hair loss is not consistent with the binge-purge cycle. It is associated with starvation and anorexia.

5. **Correct answer is a.** To interrupt the binge-purge cycle, it is necessary that clients who have bulimia be directly supervised after meals.

   b. Weighing the client too frequently reinforces the obsession with weight and food intake. Daily weigh-ins are recommended.
   c. Although providing teaching about nutrition is appropriate, this knowledge will not interrupt the compulsive cycle of bingeing and purging.
   d. During early treatment, clients who have bulimia lack the internal control to stop bingeing and purging without direct supervision. Contracts are useful as the client makes progress in treatment.

6. **Correct answer is c.** Muscle spasms are a manifestation of hypokalemia that can occur when serum potassium level has fallen below 3 mEq/L or when there has been a rapid drop in serum potassium level.

   a. Decreased bowel motility, not diarrhea, is a manifestation of hypokalemia.
   b. Since prolonged hypokalemia impairs renal functioning, dilute urine, polyuria, and nocturia occur, not urinary retention.
   d. Fatigue and low energy, not hyperactivity, accompany hypokalemia.

7. **Correct answer is c.** Because bulimic behavior is frequently a maladaptive coping mechanism in response to stress, the client must identify situations that cause the anxiety that leads to the bulimic behavior. Only then can he find alternate ways of dealing with the anxiety.

a. The client will be unable to stop his compulsive behavior simply by being given a diet to follow. Poor eating habits are not the cause of a compulsive eating disorder. Change is related to addressing underlying issues.

b. Buying large quantities of food is part of the ritual associated with bulimic behavior. It is unlikely that this compulsive behavior could be redirected without addressing underlying issues.

d. Although adaptive coping mechanisms can be learned to replace the impulse to eat, this must be done in conjunction with learning adaptive ways of dealing with the underlying causes of anxiety.

8. **Correct answer is d.** This response helps the client focus on bingeing and purging as a coping mechanism in response to emotional upset.

a. This response is punishing and does not help the client to examine his behavior.

b. This response is reassuring but does not help the client to identify the cause of his bulimic behavior.

c. This response is not appropriate because it diverts attention from the client's feelings rather than focusing on them.

9. **Correct answer is a.** Adult-onset obesity is believed to be a defense against stress.

b. Overfeeding in childhood is associated with developmental obesity.

c. Although depression can occur in clients who are obese, mood disorders are generally not associated with obesity.

d. Although obesity can occur as a result of a metabolic disorder, reactive obesity is related to psychologic issues.

11

Personality Disorders

OVERVIEW

I. General concepts
- A. Common features
- B. General symptoms
- C. Types of personality disorders
- D. Theoretic explanations of personality disorders

II. Treatments
- A. Insight-oriented psychotherapy

- B. Behavior modification
- C. Family therapy

III. Essential nursing care
- A. Nursing assessment
- B. Nursing diagnoses
- C. Planning
- D. Nursing implementation
- E. Nursing evaluation

NURSING HIGHLIGHTS

1. Providing effective nursing care to the client with a personality disorder is often problematic, because of the difficulty of establishing an honest and mutual therapeutic alliance.
2. Clients with personality disorders can provoke feelings of anger, frustration, and betrayal in caregivers; nurses caring for these clients must recognize and confront these negative emotions.
3. It is important for the nursing staff to work as a team when caring for the client with a personality disorder to avoid client attempts at manipulation.

GLOSSARY

conduct disorder—persistent pattern of behavior that violates societal rules or age-appropriate norms and the basic rights of others

countertransference—conscious or unconscious emotional response by the nurse to the behaviors of the client; response can be positive or negative

ideas of reference—the mistaken notion that outside events include important personal meanings

identity disturbance—distorted or unstable self-image or sense of self

personality trait—persistent behavioral pattern that does not significantly hinder functioning

I. General concepts

A. Common features

1. Personality disorders (PDs) primarily involve problems with interpersonal relationships.
2. PDs are generally chronic, pervasive (affecting all areas of the client's life), and maladaptive (i.e., they cause significant difficulties in living, working, and family life).
3. PDs involve exaggerations of normal personality patterns or traits.
4. PDs may coexist with other severe psychiatric problems.
5. PDs may be difficult to diagnose and treat.

B. General symptoms

1. Suspiciousness or mistrust
2. Rigid thinking
3. Distortions of reality
4. Projection
5. Restricted or exaggerated affect
6. Isolation
7. Unstable interpersonal relationships
8. Restricted or exaggerated moral development
9. Self-care deficits
10. Somatic symptoms
11. Delusional thinking
12. Poor self-esteem or excessive sense of self-importance
13. Potential for harm to self or others

C. Types of personality disorders (DSM-IV)

1. Cluster A disorders
   a) Paranoid personality disorder: a pervasive distrust of people, beginning by early adulthood, as indicated by at least 4 of the following conditions:
      (1) Suspicion, without due cause, that people are being exploitative or deceptive
      (2) Preoccupation with unjustified doubts about the loyalty or trustworthiness of one's friends or associates
      (3) Finding hidden demeaning or threatening meanings in benign remarks or events
      (4) Persistently holding grudges
      (5) Perceiving attacks (not apparent to others) on one's character or reputation, followed by a quick, angry reaction or counterattack
      (6) Recurring, unjustified suspicions that one's spouse or sexual partner is not being faithful

See text pages
_____

b) Schizoid personality disorder: a pervasive pattern of detachment from social relationships as well as a restricted range of emotional expression in interpersonal relationships, beginning by early adulthood, as indicated by at least 4 of the following symptoms:
   (1) Lack of desire for or inability to enjoy close relationships, including within one's own family
   (2) Almost exclusive preference for solitary activities
   (3) Little, if any, interest in having sexual experiences with another person
   (4) Deriving pleasure from few, if any, activities
   (5) Lack of close friends
   (6) Indifference to praise or criticism
   (7) Emotional coldness and flattened affect
c) Schizotypal personality disorder: a pervasive pattern of social and interpersonal deficits (acute discomfort with and reduced capacity for close relationships, cognitive or perceptual distortions, and eccentricities of behavior), beginning by early adulthood, as indicated by at least 5 of the following symptoms:
   (1) Ideas of reference (excluding delusions of reference)
   (2) Odd beliefs or magical thinking that influences behavior
   (3) Unusual perceptual experiences (e.g., bodily illusions)
   (4) Odd thinking and speech (e.g., vague, circumstantial, metaphorical, overelaborate, stereotypical)
   (5) Suspiciousness or paranoid thoughts
   (6) Inappropriate or constricted affect
   (7) Odd or eccentric behavior and appearance
   (8) Lack of close friends
   (9) Excessive social anxiety that does not lessen with familiarity and usually includes paranoid thoughts
2. Cluster B disorders
   a) Antisocial personality disorder
      (1) Evidence of conduct disorder before age 15 in a client at least 18 years old
      (2) A pervasive pattern of disregard for and violation of the rights of others since age 15, as indicated by at least 3 of the following conditions:
         (a) Failure to conform to social norms of lawful behavior
         (b) Irritability and aggressiveness
         (c) Irresponsibility in employment history and financial obligations
         (d) Impulsivity and failure to plan ahead
         (e) Deceitfulness

      (f) Disregard for safety of self and others

      (g) Lack of feelings of remorse

b) Borderline personality disorder: a pervasive pattern of instability in interpersonal relationships, self-image, affect, and impulse control, beginning by early adulthood, as indicated by at least 5 of the following symptoms:

    (1) Frantic efforts to avoid real or perceived abandonment (excluding suicide attempts and self-mutilating acts)

    (2) Unstable and intense personal relationships

    (3) Persistent identity disturbance

    (4) Reckless, impulsive behavior in at least 2 of the following areas: spending, sex, substance abuse, shoplifting, driving, binge eating

    (5) Recurrent suicidal behavior or gestures or threats or self-mutilating acts

    (6) Marked reactivity of moods, usually lasting for short periods and rarely more than a few days

    (7) Chronic feelings of emptiness or boredom

    (8) Inappropriate, intense anger; lack of anger control

    (9) Transient, stress-related paranoid thoughts or severe dissociative symptoms

c) Histrionic personality disorder: a pervasive pattern of excessive emotionality and attention-seeking behavior, beginning by early adulthood, as indicated by at least 5 of the following symptoms:

    (1) Feeling uncomfortable when one is not the center of attention

    (2) Inappropriately sexually seductive in behavior or appearance

    (3) Labile emotions

    (4) Overly concerned with physical appearance, using it to draw attention to oneself

    (5) Style of speech that is excessively impressionistic and lacking in details

    (6) Self-dramatization, theatricality, and exaggerated expression of emotion

    (7) Suggestibility

    (8) Mistaken belief that one's relationships with others are more intimate than they actually are

d) Narcissistic personality disorder: a pervasive pattern of grandiosity, need for admiration, and lack of empathy, beginning in early adulthood, as indicated by at least 5 of the following symptoms:

    (1) Strong sense of self-importance

    (2) Preoccupation with thoughts of unlimited success, beauty, intelligence, power, or love

    (3) Belief that one is superior and should associate only with other superior people or institutions

    (4) Need for excessive admiration and attention

    (5) Strong sense of being entitled to special treatment

    (6) Exploitation of others

    (7) Lack of empathy

        (8) Envy of others or belief that others envy him/her

        (9) Arrogant behaviors and attitudes

3. Cluster C disorders

   a) Avoidant personality disorder: a pervasive pattern of social inhibition, feelings of inadequacy, and hypersensitivity to criticism, beginning in adulthood, as indicated by at least 4 of the following symptoms:

      (1) Avoidance of occupational activities involving significant interpersonal contact

      (2) Unwillingness to risk getting involved in relationships without being certain of succeeding in being liked

      (3) Restraint within intimate relationships

      (4) Preoccupation with fears of being rejected or criticized in social situations

      (5) Inhibition within new relationships

      (6) Belief that one is socially inept, personally unappealing, or inferior to others

      (7) Unwillingness to take personal risks or engage in new activities

   b) Dependent personality disorder: a pervasive and excessive need to be taken care of, leading to submissive and clinging behaviors and fears of separation, beginning in early adulthood, as indicated by at least 5 of the following symptoms:

      (1) Inability to make everyday decisions without excessive advice from others

      (2) Need for others to take over important responsibilities in one's life

      (3) Reluctance to disagree with others because of fear of being rejected

      (4) Difficulty initiating projects and doing things on one's own

      (5) Extraordinary attempts to get emotional support from others (e.g., volunteering to do unpleasant things)

      (6) Feeling uncomfortable or helpless when alone

      (7) Attempting to find a new dependent relationship when a close relationship ends

      (8) Preoccupation with fears of being left alone to care for oneself

   c) Obsessive-compulsive personality disorder: a pervasive pattern of preoccupation with orderliness, perfectionism, and mental and interpersonal control at the expense of flexibility, openness, and efficiency, beginning by early adulthood, as indicated by at least 4 of the following symptoms:

      (1) Preoccupation with details, rules, lists, organization, or schedules, causing inability to focus on the main point of the activity

      (2) Perfectionism that interferes with task completion

(3) Excessive devotion to work and productivity with exclusion of leisure activities and friendships

(4) Overconscientiousness, scrupulousness, and inflexibility regarding morality, ethics, or values

(5) Inability to discard worthless objects

(6) Reluctance to delegate tasks unless work will be done exactly as he/she would do it

(7) Miserliness with money

(8) Rigidity and stubbornness

d) Passive-aggressive personality

(1) Listed separately as a cluster C disorder in DSM-III-R; in DSM-IV, listed as a nonspecific personality disorder that has behaviors of more than 1 personality disorder but not full criteria for any 1 personality disorder

(2) General symptoms of passive-aggressive behavior affecting social and job interactions

(a) Procrastination

(b) Failure to do job or doing poor job when work is something one doesn't want to do

(c) Resentment of suggestions about how to improve performance

(d) Failure to do fair share of work

(e) Excessively scornful and critical of people in authority

(f) Claims that demands made on him/her are unreasonable and irritability and argumentativeness when asked to perform a task

D. Theoretic explanations of personality disorders

1. Biologic influences

2. Social and environmental influences

3. Family influences

4. Reinforcement of behavioral responses

II. Treatments

A. Insight-oriented psychotherapy

B. Behavior modification

C. Family therapy

See text pages
_____

III. Essential nursing care

A. Nursing assessment

1. Take histories.

a) Medical

b) Psychiatric

c) Family

d) Social

e) Current problems

See text pages
_____

2. Assess current mental status: Record observations of client's behavior, affect, and interaction.
3. Assess coping mechanisms: Identify constructive and destructive coping mechanisms.
4. Assess altered thought processes.
5. Assess social interaction.
6. Evaluate for symptoms of personality disorders.

B. Nursing diagnoses
   1. Main NANDA nursing diagnoses
      a) Ineffective individual coping
      b) Social isolation
   2. Additional NANDA nursing diagnoses
      a) Impaired adjustment
      b) Anxiety
      c) High risk for violence, self-directed or directed at others
      d) Ineffective family coping
      e) Impaired social interaction
      f) Self-care deficit
      g) Self-esteem disturbance
   3. Selected complete nursing diagnoses
      a) Ineffective individual coping related to difficulty in maintaining interpersonal relationships evidenced by statement that "all my friends have let me down"
      b) Social isolation related to antisocial behavior evidenced by lack of significant others identified in nursing assessment
      c) Ineffective family coping related to client's social detachment evidenced by conflicts over family rules

C. Planning (goal setting)
   1. General goals
      a) Establish therapeutic alliance.
      b) Reduce impairments of perception.
      c) Assist in development and maintenance of healthy, positive, and self-enhancing relationships with others.
      d) Promote healthy activities, and reduce anxiety.
      e) Maintain biologic integrity.
   2. Examples of specific goals
      a) Client will express anger without physical violence.
      b) Client will express the desire to establish new friendships.

D. Nursing implementation (intervention)
   1. General interventions for personality disorders
      a) Establish therapeutic alliance.
         (1) Respect client's privacy.

    (2) Establish consistency.
        (a) Assigning same caregivers can help ensure that consistent messages are given.
        (b) Setting consistent limits can decrease the possibility that client will be able to manipulate staff.
    (3) Give positive reinforcement in a matter-of-fact manner.
    (4) Deal with client honestly.
    (5) Implement behavior modification interventions established in the treatment plan.
    (6) Promote clear, consistent, and open communication.
  b) Reduce impairments of perception.
    (1) When client expresses distortions of reality, acknowledge client's feelings while stating that you do not share his/her interpretation of events.
    (2) Refocus client interactions on reality rather than on perceived threats or slights.
    (3) Point out inconsistent behavior.
    (4) Use specific and concrete words.
    (5) Provide feedback and insight about specific dysfunctional personality features (e.g., passivity, dependence, or obsessiveness).
  c) Assist in development of healthy and positive relationships with others.
    (1) Introduce client to group situations.
    (2) Help client examine how his/her behavior precipitated the current crisis.
  d) Promote healthy activities, and reduce anxiety.
    (1) Help client to participate in diversionary and stress-relieving activities (e.g., leisure activities or exercise).
    (2) Use role-playing techniques to help client identify maladaptive thoughts and behaviors.
    (3) Provide a structured environment (daily schedule of activities).
  e) Maintain biologic integrity.
    (1) Assist client in developing schedules and goals for basic self-care activities.
    (2) Monitor client who is at risk for self-destructive behavior.
    (3) Make appropriate referrals to community agencies.
2. Specific interventions for cluster A personality disorders
  a) With paranoid client, remain calm and nonthreatening.
  b) Have client with schizoid or schizotypal disorder participate in group activities.
3. Specific interventions for cluster B personality disorders
  a) Avoid falling prey to attempts at manipulation by client with antisocial personality disorder (see Nurse Alert, "Intervening in Manipulative Behavior").
  b) Establish clear guidelines for behavior with client with borderline personality disorder.

      c) Avoid paying attention to sexually provocative behaviors of client with histrionic personality disorder.

      d) Help client with narcissistic personality disorder to acknowledge the rights and needs of others.

    4. Specific interventions for cluster C personality disorders

      a) Help the client with avoidant personality disorder to develop self-esteem and form relationships.

      b) Encourage the client with dependent personality disorder to recognize strengths and abilities.

      c) Help the client with obsessive-compulsive personality disorder to participate in pleasurable activities.

      d) Encourage the client with passive-aggressive personality disorder to identify direct ways of expressing feelings.

E. Nursing evaluation

  1. Evaluation of goal achievement is ongoing; goals and care plan are revised as needed.

  2. If goals were not achieved, assess reasons.

    a) Were goals realistic?

    b) Were problems identified correctly?

    c) Was enough time allowed for achievement of goals?

  3. Keep in mind that progress toward goals is usually slow for clients with personality disorders, due to the chronicity of the problem, the well-developed defenses, the difficulties in establishing a therapeutic alliance, and the often short duration of therapy.

! NURSE *ALERT* !

Intervening in Manipulative Behavior

- Set limits on behavior.
  - —Specify behaviors that will not be tolerated.
  - —Enforce limits consistently.
- Help client to gain self-control over unacceptable manipulative behaviors.
  - —Identify alternative way to obtain needs.
  - —Use behavior modification techniques (e.g., contracts).
  - —Help client identify feelings.
- Do not allow countertransference to interfere with therapeutic alliance.
  - —Avoid getting into power struggles or arguments.
  - —Maintain a matter-of-fact demeanor.
- Make decisions in a group setting, because a group is more difficult to manipulate than an individual nurse.

1. Elaine, a client who has borderline personality disorder, is admitted to the psychiatric unit following a suicide attempt. During the nursing assessment, she states to her primary nurse, "I've never met anyone as smart as you. I wish I could be like you." The nurse recognizes in these statements the primitive defense mechanism of:

   a. Depersonalization.
   b. Splitting.
   c. Omnipotence.
   d. Denial.

2. In the morning, Elaine sleeps through the community meeting. When approached by her primary nurse about the absence, Elaine begins crying and screams, "You hate me, and you are out to get me in trouble." The best response by the nurse is:

   a. "Why are you so angry?"
   b. "All the clients attend community meeting daily."
   c. "I'm sorry I upset you."
   d. "Try to come tomorrow if you can."

3. Arnold was admitted for inpatient treatment when he became depressed following the death of his mother. Along with the depression, Arnold has been diagnosed with schizoid personality disorder. An appropriate nursing diagnosis for schizoid personality disorder is:

   a. Social isolation.
   b. Powerlessness.
   c. Potential for violence, self-directed.
   d. Altered thought processes.

4. When assessing the cognitive function of a client who has schizotypal personality disorder, the nurse would most likely find:

   a. Abstract thinking.
   b. Obsessions.
   c. Auditory hallucinations.
   d. Magical thinking.

5. The nursing diagnosis of anxiety related to social situations in the client with a diagnosis of schizotypal personality disorder is frequently accompanied by which of the following symptoms?

   a. Aggressive behavior
   b. Depression
   c. Paranoid thoughts
   d. Low self-esteem

6. Nelson, age 23, was sent by the court to a community mental health center for evaluation after he assaulted his mother. His mother stated to the court, "Nelson beat me up because I would not let him borrow my car." Which of the following reactions by Nelson is consistent with antisocial personality disorder?

   a. Nelson is tearful and upset about the incident.
   b. Nelson is angry and blames his mother for the incident.
   c. Nelson is quiet and withdrawn.
   d. Nelson is experiencing auditory hallucinations.

7. Nelson's antisocial behavior demonstrates a severe problem with:

   a. Dependency needs.
   b. Development of conscience.
   c. Sexual identity.
   d. Restricted affect.

8. The nurse identifies a nursing diagnosis of impaired social interaction for a client with a diagnosis of narcissistic personality disorder. Which of the following behaviors would the client exhibit?

   a. Arrogance and attempts at exploitation
   b. Social withdrawal
   c. Avoidance of sexual interaction
   d. Eccentric and inappropriate speech

9. Ineffective individual coping in a client with a diagnosis of dependent personality disorder is most likely to be evidenced by:

   a. Fear of becoming involved in a significant relationship.
   b. Preference for solitary activities.
   c. Recurrent suicidal behavior.
   d. Inability to make decisions without advice.

10. When planning care for the client with a diagnosis of obsessive-compulsive personality disorder, the nurse recognizes that the client's defenses are most likely maintained by:

   a. Somatic symptoms.
   b. Rules and orderliness.
   c. Arrogant behaviors.
   d. Dependent behaviors.

11. Which of the following is an appropriate nursing care goal for the client with a diagnosis of obsessive-compulsive personality disorder?

   a. Client will participate in pleasurable activities.
   b. Client will arrive at group therapy on time.
   c. Client will assume responsibility for work.
   d. Client will reduce impulsive behavior.

12. When the nurse is implementing care for the manipulative client, the priority is to:

   a. Be consistent and firm.
   b. Use negative reinforcement.
   c. Remain flexible.
   d. Avoid angry interactions.

ANSWERS

1. **Correct answer is b.** In splitting, the client sees herself or others as either all good (idealized) or all bad (devalued).

   a. Depersonalization is experienced by the client with borderline personality disorder as a feeling of loss of normal sense of self.
   c. Omnipotence is manifested as feelings of power and superiority over others.

   d. Denial is a defense mechanism that manifests as a refusal to acknowledge feelings.

2. **Correct answer is b.** Clients with a diagnosis of borderline personality disorder require structure. The nurse's statement that everyone attends the community meeting daily sets a limit and clarifies for the client that she will not be given special treatment.

   a. Clients with borderline personality disorder usually do not recognize the source of their anger.
   c. It is nontherapeutic for the nurse to apologize. The nurse must recognize that the client will experience anger when expectations for appropriate behavior are identified.
   d. This response is nontherapeutic because it does not provide structure. Lack of clear directions and limits increases the anxiety and acting-out behavior.

3. **Correct answer is a.** Characteristic of the client with schizoid personality disorder are the inability to form close relationships and a preference for solitary activities.

   b. Powerlessness is not usually identified among clients with schizoid personality disorder. They are emotionally indifferent.
   c. Although potential for self-directed violence may occur in connection with depression, generally it is not characteristic of the schizoid personality disorder.
   d. Although clients with schizoid personality disorder have a restricted emotional range, there is no evidence of altered thought processes.

4. **Correct answer is d.** Clients who have schizotypal personality disorder experience cognitive disturbances, including magical thinking and ideas of reference.

   a. The client with a diagnosis of schizotypal personality disorder demonstrates concrete, not abstract, thinking.
   b. Obsessions are not characteristic of the cognitive functioning of the client with a diagnosis of schizotypal personality disorder.

c. Although clients with schizotypal personality disorder exhibit oddities of thought, perception, speech, and behavior, they do not experience auditory hallucinations.

5. **Correct answer is c.** Clients with schizotypal personality disorder experience excessive social anxiety that can lead to paranoid thoughts.

   a. Although agitation can occur with severe anxiety, the client with a diagnosis of schizotypal personality disorder usually does not become aggressive.
   b. Constricted affect in the client with a diagnosis of schizotypal personality disorder may be mistaken for depression. However, affective symptoms usually are not noted in response to social anxiety.
   d. Although self-esteem may be an underlying issue, it is difficult to evaluate in clients with schizotypal personality disorder. Cognitive distortions and eccentric behaviors are dominant characteristics.

6. **Correct answer is b.** A client with a diagnosis of antisocial personality disorder feels neither remorse nor responsibility for his actions. He blames others for his behavior.

   a. Feelings of remorse and guilt are atypical of antisocial personality disorder.
   c. Clients with antisocial personality disorder are usually angry and impulsive when confronted with their inappropriate actions, not quiet and withdrawn.
   d. Clients with antisocial personality disorder usually do not exhibit psychotic symptoms.

7. **Correct answer is b.** The key feature of antisocial personality disorder is failure to develop a conscience, leading to lack of guilt about improper behavior.

   a. Clients with antisocial personality disorder have not developed the emotional bonds that would cause them to struggle with dependency needs.
   c. Although clients with antisocial personality disorder may experience sexual identity

conflicts, generally the cause of their acting-out behavior is related to impulsiveness and failure to acquire social values.
d. Rather than demonstrating a restricted affect, clients with antisocial personality disorder are impulsive and often irritable and aggressive.

8. **Correct answer is a.** The client with a diagnosis of narcissistic personality disorder has difficulty maintaining lasting relationships due to superior attitude and using others to gain attention and admiration.

   b. Clients with narcissistic personality disorder seek attention and admiration.
   c. Clients with narcissistic personality disorder often are promiscuous.
   d. Eccentric and inappropriate speech is a characteristic of schizotypal personality disorder, not narcissistic personality disorder.

9. **Correct answer is d.** Indecisiveness is typical of dependent personality disorder. Clients with this disorder act out submissive and clinging behaviors so that others will make decisions for them.

   a. The client with a diagnosis of dependent personality disorder pursues relationships in order to be taken care of.
   b. The client with a diagnosis of dependent personality disorder feels helpless and uncomfortable when alone. Solitary activities are avoided.
   c. Although a client with a diagnosis of dependent personality disorder may become depressed and suicidal if needs are not met, this is not a typical response.

10. **Correct answer is b.** Preoccupation with details, rules, lists, organization, and schedules is typical of the client with a diagnosis of obsessive-compulsive personality disorder.

    a. Somatic symptoms are not typical of the client with obsessive-compulsive personality disorder.
    c. Arrogant behavior is not typical of the client with obsessive-compulsive personality disorder. Affect tends to be restricted.

d. Clients with obsessive-compulsive personality disorder do not form dependent relationships. An excessive devotion to work and productivity usually excludes close relationships.

11. **Correct answer is a.** Clients with a diagnosis of obsessive-compulsive personality disorder usually forgo pleasurable activities in order to give attention to work, organization, and details. Experiencing a pleasurable activity represents growth and change.

    b. This is not an appropriate nursing goal, since clients with a diagnosis of obsessive-compulsive personality disorder are usually punctual.

    c. This is not an appropriate nursing goal, since clients with a diagnosis of obsessive-compulsive personality disorder are usually devoted to work.

d. This is not an appropriate nursing goal, since clients with obsessive-compulsive personality disorder do not demonstrate impulsive behavior; they exhibit rigidity.

12. **Correct answer is a.** Consistency helps reduce the manipulative client's anxiety and builds trust in the client.

    b. Using negative reinforcement does not identify acceptable behaviors for the manipulative client and diminishes the client's self-esteem.

    c. Flexibility encourages manipulative clients to make further attempts to control situations.

    d. When the nurse sets limits on a manipulative client, anger is an expected outcome. Manipulative clients must learn to tolerate unpleasant feelings.

12

Special Populations and Issues

NURSING HIGHLIGHTS

1. Nurses providing psychiatric nursing care encounter a variety of special populations, each of which requires a flexible approach and sensitivity to specific issues.
2. Many nonpsychiatric problems—such as HIV (human immunodeficiency virus) infection and abuse—include a psychiatric dimension.
3. The practice of psychiatric nursing involves important legal and ethical responsibilities.

GLOSSARY

commitment—involuntary admission to a psychiatric facility; the legal process by which a person is involuntarily admitted to a facility
dyspareunia—pain occurring with sexual intercourse
frotteurism—sexual arousal resulting from fantasies or acts involving rubbing against a nonconsenting individual
paraphilia—sexual disorder in which sexual arousal is achieved in response to objects or situations that are bizarre or unnatural

primary depression—feelings of sadness that are not in reaction to a precipitating event (e.g., death of a loved one)

secondary depression—feelings of sadness that occur in response to a precipitating event (e.g., death of a loved one)

vaginismus—sexual disorder involving involuntary spasms of the vaginal muscles, which prevent sexual intercourse

ENHANCED OUTLINE

I. Clients with HIV/AIDS

See text pages

A. Mental health concerns
  1. HIV dementia complex (HIV encephalopathy)
     a) HIV virus acts directly on brain tissue.
     b) Symptoms include forgetfulness, decreased concentration, confusion, loss of balance, muscle weakness, decreased sexual urges, deterioration in fine motor skills, depression, apathy, and withdrawal.
     c) Symptoms are generally not responsive to counseling or other treatments.
  2. Anxiety and depression (see Chapters 5 and 7)
     a) Feelings of depression and anxiety are secondary symptoms that result from extensive losses experienced by person with HIV or AIDS.
     b) Losses occur in the areas of energy, physical strength, cognitive ability, financial security, physical appearance, physical intimacy, and life.
     c) These secondary symptoms may be difficult to distinguish from primary dementia but may respond to counseling or other interventions.

B. Nursing considerations
  1. Promote physical comfort.
  2. Maintain the client's dignity.
  3. Assist the client in working through the stages of grief.
  4. Support the family and significant others.
  5. Address staff issues.
     a) Rotate staff regularly to help prevent burnout.
     b) Encourage the expression of feelings.
     c) Provide education about HIV and AIDS, including methods of transmission and the impact on caregivers.

II. Children and adolescents

See text pages

A. Mental health concerns
  1. Social and cultural factors: physical environment (home and community), family dynamics, socioeconomic level, and social supports

2. Psychiatric disorders common among children
   a) Disruptive behavior disorders: attention deficit–hyperactivity disorder, conduct disorder, and oppositional defiant disorder
   b) Separation anxiety disorder
   c) Pervasive developmental disorders: autism (impaired interpersonal skills as well as motor manifestations, such as spinning, flapping of arms, and body rocking)
   d) Mood disorders: primary and secondary depressions
   e) Tic disorders: grimacing, eye blinking or squinting, squatting, hopping, or vocalizing (grunting, barking, stuttering, or uttering obscene words and phrases)
3. Psychiatric disorders common among adolescents
   a) Identity disorder
      (1) Adolescent feels distress and has difficulty forming his/her identity (e.g., regarding career choices, moral values, and sexual role).
      (2) This disorder must be distinguished from normal developmental issues.
   b) Adjustment disorder: Child demonstrates a maladaptive response to a psychosocial stressor (e.g., divorce of parents).
   c) Depression and suicide: Occurrences are epidemic among adolescents and children (see Chapter 7).
   d) Substance abuse (see Chapter 9)
   e) Eating disorders (see Chapter 10)

B. Nursing considerations
   1. Make age-appropriate assessment, taking into account normal developmental schedule.
   2. Use appropriate assessment tools, including play, drawings, observation, and interview.
   3. Perform family assessment, including factors such as the family's commitment to the child, intimacy, problem-solving ability, and social and communication skills.

III. Elderly clients

A. Mental health concerns
   1. Age-related psychologic changes: Normal age-related psychologic changes (decreases in memory and in problem-solving, learning, and coping abilities) must be differentiated from abnormal changes.
   2. Psychiatric problems common among the elderly
      a) Depression and suicide (see Chapter 7)
      b) Cognitive disorders: delirium (same as Chapter 8, section II) and dementia (same as Chapter 8, section III)
      c) Substance abuse (see Chapter 9)
      d) Delusional disorder (see Chapter 6, section I,A,2,b,1 and section I,D,3)

B. Nursing considerations
   1. Take into account the physiologic and psychologic effects of aging (e.g., visual and hearing losses mimicking confusion, slowed response times, and short-term memory impairment) when making assessments.

See text pages _____

I. Clients with HIV/AIDS	II. Children and adolescents	III. Elderly clients	IV. Victims of violence and abuse	V. Sexual disorders

2. Tailor interventions to the elderly client (e.g., allow more time for communication, observe for fatigue, and be aware of possible reluctance to discuss intimate matters and client's preconceptions of nurses' and physicians' roles).
3. Distinguish symptoms of depression from those of dementia (see Nurse Alert in Chapter 8, "How to Differentiate between Dementia and Depression among the Elderly").

See text pages

_____

IV. Victims of violence and abuse

A. Children
   1. Background
      a) Child abuse occurs in all cultural groups and at all socioeconomic levels.
      b) Child abuse can involve neglect and physical, sexual, psychologic, and/or emotional abuse.
      c) Risk factors for committing child abuse may or may not be apparent.
         (1) A history of being abused
         (2) Inadequate coping skills
         (3) Inadequate parenting skills
         (4) Social isolation
         (5) Authoritarian or harsh parenting style
   2. Nursing considerations
      a) Be alert to the possibility of child abuse in all practice settings.
      b) Exercise the legal obligation to report abuse or suspected abuse.
      c) Maintain objectivity when treating victims of child abuse to ensure effective nursing care.
      d) Make referrals to appropriate agencies for follow-up care and placement.

B. Adults
   1. Background
      a) Adult victims of abuse are often in positions of powerlessness (e.g., the mentally retarded, the elderly, and women).
      b) Victims of chronic abuse may be in a dependent relationship with the abuser, creating conflicted emotions and impeding effective action to end the abuse.
      c) Victims of sexual assault may experience rape-trauma syndrome, a severe psychologic reaction with both acute and delayed phases (see Nurse Alert, "Phases of Rape-Trauma Syndrome").
   2. Nursing considerations: Nursing care is generally supportive.
      a) Serve as a referral source.
      b) Help the client verbalize the abusive experience.

Phases of Rape-Trauma Syndrome

Phase	Reactions
• Acute phase	• Emotional: fear, shock, anxiety, humiliation, denial, helplessness, self-blame
	• Physical: vaginal trauma, bruises, soreness, headaches, sleep disturbances, gastrointestinal dysfunction
• Outward adjustment phase	• Outward calmness masking feelings of shock, disbelief, and numbness
• Reorganization phase	• Phobias, sexual dysfunctions, strong urge to discuss rape, nightmares, insomnia, crying spells, depression

    c) Document and collect physical evidence of rape or other form of abuse. (Nurses must be familiar with state legal requirements for collecting and maintaining custody of forensic evidence.)

V. Sexual disorders

A. Background

    1. A variety of "nonstandard" sexual behaviors may be encountered, but they are not necessarily disorders.

    2. The definition of a sexual disorder is somewhat imprecise: Sexual behaviors are classified as sexual disorders when they are maladaptive for the client, pose a threat of harm to the client or others, or lessen the client's ability to develop close relationships.

        a) Sexual desire disorders: hypoactive sexual desire disorder, sexual aversion disorder

        b) Sexual arousal disorders: female sexual arousal disorder, male erectile disorder

        c) Orgasm disorders: female orgasmic disorder, male orgasmic disorder, premature ejaculation

        d) Sexual pain disorders: dyspareunia, vaginismus

        e) Paraphilias: exhibitionism, fetishism, frotteurism, pedophilia, sexual masochism, sexual sadism, voyeurism, transvestic fetishism

        f) Gender identity disorder

B. Nursing considerations

    1. Implement behavior therapy techniques as described in treatment plan.

    2. Provide information on nonproblematic sexual behaviors.

    3. Promote more effective patterns of sexuality.

    4. Reduce anxiety about sexual problems.

VI. Legal/ethical issues

A. Hospitalization/discharge

    1. Hospitalization

        a) Voluntary admission: Client requests admission and has the right to be released upon request.

See text pages

See text pages

  b) Involuntary hospitalization: 1 or more of the following criteria are necessary.
    (1) Client is a danger to self or others.
    (2) Client is unable to meet basic self-care needs.
    (3) Client is mentally ill.
 2. Discharge
  a) Conditional discharge: Certain conditions must be fulfilled, or client will be hospitalized again.
    (1) Fulfilling outpatient treatment requirements
    (2) Meeting basic self-care needs
    (3) Complying with medication schedules
  b) Absolute discharge: Client is released from hospital unconditionally.

B. Client rights
 1. Right to accept or refuse treatment, except in cases of civil commitment or criminal conviction
 2. Right to due process of law in cases of civil commitment
 3. Right to least restrictive alternative: Provide adequate care to protect client and others from harm while allowing maximum freedom.
 4. Right to informed consent: Treatment must be explained, including reasons for it, risks and benefits, alternatives, probability of success, and likely outcomes if treatment is declined.

C. Nursing responsibilities
 1. Nurses have a duty to preserve client confidentiality except when this duty conflicts with the nurses' responsibility to report elder/child abuse or to warn third parties who may be in danger because of a client.
 2. Nurses have a duty to provide care.
 3. Nurses have a duty to keep accurate and complete medical records.

D. Liability
 1. Nurses can be held liable for nursing malpractice (i.e., the failure to perform according to generally accepted standards in client care).
 2. Complete and accurate documentation (charting) is the best protection against liability. (See Chapter 4, section VII, for the proper methods of recording information.)

E. Advocacy: Nurses can serve as advocates for psychiatric clients through a number of activities.
 1. Providing accurate information to the public at large
 2. Providing testimony and input on policy decisions
 3. Securing access to community resources and making referrals to inform clients of their options

1. Mr. Adams, who is HIV positive, was recently admitted to the psychiatric unit of a hospital. Mr. Bledsoe, another client on the unit, comes to the nurse and says, "We hear that guy has AIDS, and we want him out of here." Which response by the nurse is most appropriate?

   a. "It is not true that Mr. Adams has AIDS."
   b. "Information about other clients is confidential; I cannot discuss this with you."
   c. "What exactly do you know about HIV and AIDS?"
   d. "Only the doctor can discharge clients; you should talk with him."

2. Sam, age 7, has a diagnosis of attention deficit–hyperactivity disorder (ADHD). Which combination of treatments would be most beneficial to him?

   a. Methylphenidate hydrochloride (Ritalin) and sympathy
   b. Chlorpromazine (Thorazine) and structure
   c. Methylphenidate hydrochloride and structure
   d. Chlorpromazine and sympathy

3. If Sam straightens up his room on a particular day, which of the following comments should the nurse suggest that Sam's mother make to encourage him to do it again?

   a. "You're a good boy, Sam."
   b. "Now that you can pick up your room, be sure to do it tomorrow."
   c. "What a pretty room you have."
   d. "I like it that you picked up your room."

4. Mrs. DeVito, age 89, has been admitted to the nursing unit with symptoms of forgetfulness and inability to make decisions and to concentrate. The nurse would expect which of the following to be the initial step taken by the treatment team?

   a. Psychotherapy to decrease anxiety
   b. Antidepressants to improve memory
   c. Careful diagnostic studies
   d. Attention to nutrition and hygiene

5. Mrs. DeVito's illness is diagnosed as dementia of the Alzheimer's type. Which statement made by Mrs. DeVito's daughter indicates that the daughter understands the family education provided by the nurse?

   a. "No one really knows why this happened to my mother."
   b. "This is a natural part of aging."
   c. "Nothing can help Mother now."
   d. "I told Mother to slow down or she would go crazy."

6. A 20-year-old housewife comes to the clinic with multiple body bruises that are partially healed, swelling around both eyes, and a handprint-shaped bruise on her cheek. She seems timid and evasive and reports that she fell down the stairs. While the nurse is alone with the client in the examination room, which action is appropriate?

   a. Say nothing until the client volunteers that she has been abused.
   b. Ask the client if someone has caused these injuries.
   c. Tell the client to leave her husband's house immediately.
   d. Call the police to report the findings and suspicions.

7. Mrs. Tunney discusses her husband's condition with the nurse. His wife explains that Mr. Tunney is depressed but refuses to seek medical or psychiatric help. Which statement by Mrs. Tunney would most likely indicate that it is necessary to admit Mr. Tunney to a psychiatric hospital involuntarily?

   a. "He just sits around the house all day and doesn't do anything."
   b. "He says that he would be better off dead, and I think he has some pills."
   c. "He is so cross and irritable with our children that they don't want to come home."
   d. "I can't go on much longer if I don't get something done about him."

8. Mr. Tunney is admitted to the hospital involuntarily. Once there, he refuses to participate in his treatment and refuses all medications, saying, "It's no use; it will just prolong the agony." Which principle should guide the health care team's approach?

 a. Even though Mr. Tunney was admitted involuntarily, he still retains the right to refuse treatment, and a separate court action must be sought.

 b. Because Mr. Tunney was admitted involuntarily, the staff can medicate him against his wishes if the medication is necessary to his treatment.

 c. The health care team can request that Mrs. Tunney, as Mr. Tunney's next of kin, sign a consent to administer medications to Mr. Tunney whether he refuses or not.

 d. If the physician orders medication for Mr. Tunney, the nurses have a responsibility to administer it by whatever means necessary.

ANSWERS

1. **Correct answer is c.** The nurse cannot disclose confidential information about 1 client to another client. By asking this question, the nurse can assess what Mr. Blake knows about AIDS and HIV and whether he would benefit from health teaching on these topics. The nurse can also allow Mr. Blake to ventilate without conveying confidential information to him.

 a. The nurse cannot disclose any information about a client, whether the information is positive or negative. Although the statement by the nurse that Mr. Adams does not have AIDS is technically true, it is misleading. It violates the trust she may have established with Mr. Blake, as well as violating Mr. Adams's right to confidentiality.
 b. This is a true statement, and the nurse may have to say this if Mr. Blake is persistent. This is not the best choice for an initial response, since it would tend to cut off communication.

 d. It is true that the physician is responsible for discharge. However, this response by the nurse is not appropriate; it does not help to resolve Mr. Blake's concerns or to educate him about HIV and AIDS.

2. **Correct answer is c.** Children with a diagnosis of ADHD may benefit from stimulants such as methylphenidate hydrochloride. These drugs are thought to act by stimulating the centers in the brain that inhibit impulses. These children also respond to a structured, stable environment and to behavior modification.

 a. Children with a diagnosis of ADHD may benefit from methylphenidate hydrochloride, but they do not need sympathy (especially the sort of sympathy that tolerates unacceptable behavior). Instead, they need empathy and a structured environment.
 b and d. Neuroleptic drugs such as chlorpromazine are not usually effective in controlling the behavior of children with a diagnosis of ADHD.

3. **Correct answer is d.** Immediate and specific positive reinforcement is most likely to encourage repeated behavior.

 a. Positive and negative reinforcement should center on the behavior, not on the child. General comments, such as "You're a good boy," do not give the child enough information about what he has done that is acceptable or unacceptable.
 b. This comment does not reward Sam for his behavior; it merely sets new expectations.
 c. This comment does not tell Sam what he has done; it does not reinforce the desired behavior.

4. **Correct answer is c.** Mrs. DeVito needs a careful diagnostic evaluation to establish the cause of her symptoms. Many conditions (e.g., dementia, depression, malnutrition, infection, and dehydration) produce these symptoms.

 a. These symptoms might be present with moderate levels of anxiety, but it is important to be sure of the cause before prescribing treatment.

b. If depression is present, antidepressants will often alleviate the symptoms and improve the client's quality of life dramatically. However, the first step must be a clear diagnosis.

d. There are no data to indicate that Mrs. DeVito needs assistance in these areas. Nutrition and hygiene should be assessed along with other indicators of her general health status before the treatment plan is completed.

5. **Correct answer is a.** Although theories of causation are being developed for dementia of the Alzheimer's type, the etiology has not been established.

b. Dementia is not a normal, inevitable part of aging.

c. Although there is no cure for Alzheimer's disease, medical and nursing measures can promote a more comfortable and satisfactory lifestyle. For example, neuroleptic drugs may help control agitation or insomnia, and providing a structured, predictable environment may help the client compensate for memory loss.

d. There is no evidence that stress predisposes a client to dementia.

6. **Correct answer is b.** A direct, neutral question asked in the privacy of the examination room may elicit information about possible abuse. A question of this kind should never be asked in the presence of someone else, nor should the nurse insist on an answer.

a. Because clients who have been abused often have low self-esteem and may feel that the abuse is somehow "deserved," they may be too frightened to volunteer information. The nurse needs to take the initiative in creating a climate in which the client can feel free to discuss her situation. Suspected spousal abuse must never be ignored.

c. This response would be inappropriate without further assessment.

d. This approach is not warranted until the client has had a chance to tell her story; in many clinics, a call to the police would require a team or administrative decision.

7. **Correct answer is b.** Suicidal statements plus a means for suicide indicate that the client may be dangerous to himself; this is a reason for involuntary treatment in almost every jurisdiction.

a, c, and **d.** These behaviors are symptomatic of depression or a physical problem and indicate that the client needs help, but they are not sufficient legal justification for involuntary treatment.

8. **Correct answer is a.** Involuntary admission does not remove the client's right to refuse specific treatments unless a life-threatening emergency exists. If Mr. Tunney persists in refusal of all treatment options, the treatment team will need to seek further direction from the court.

b. Clients who are admitted involuntarily retain all other civil rights, unless these have been specifically addressed by the court.

c. Before Mrs. Tunney can sign a consent directing staff to administer medication against Mr. Tunney's wishes, Mr. Tunney must be shown to be incompetent, or a life-threatening emergency must exist.

d. Mr. Tunney's right to refuse medication overrides the physician's medication order; the nurses could be liable for having administered the medication under those circumstances.

Psychiatric Nursing Comprehensive Review Questions

1. Therapeutic communication must include which of the following 3 qualities?

   a. Honesty, redundancy, rigidity
   b. Efficiency, flexibility, appropriateness
   c. Selectivity, clarity, receptivity
   d. Engagement, fluidity, eloquence

2. Which of the following statements reflects a basic principle of family therapy?

   a. The symptoms of the individual family members are an expression of family pathology.
   b. Family therapy helps the family members learn new ways of coping with the identified client.
   c. Family therapy aims to explore the intrapsychic function of each individual family member.
   d. All registered nurses do family therapy in their daily practice.

3. Ms. Lark has been hospitalized for a depression not relieved by medications and for persistent suicidal ideation. Electroconvulsive therapy (ECT) is planned. Ms. Lark says, "I'm really scared. I saw a movie once, and it was awful." The nurse should:

   a. Explain that modern ECT is much more comfortable for the client.
   b. Assure her that there is no danger.
   c. Explain the importance of complying with the suggestions of her doctor.
   d. Find out exactly what the client saw.

4. Which question by the nurse is likely to elicit the most data for evaluating a client's judgment and reasoning ability?

   a. "What day of the week is this?"
   b. "Who is the President of the United States?"
   c. "How have you been feeling lately?"
   d. "What would you do if you found a letter with a stamp?"

5. In order to evaluate Mr. Jacobs, the nurse uses the serial 7s test. When Mr. Jacobs is unable to perform the test, the nurse recognizes difficulty with:

   a. Concentration.
   b. Reality orientation.
   c. Memory.
   d. Speech patterns.

6. A client who has obsessive-compulsive disorder asks the nurse, "How can I keep from worrying that an intruder is going to break in? I check my locks a hundred times a day." Which response by the nurse reflects an approach that has been effective in helping clients interrupt obsessive thinking and compulsive behavior?

   a. "Wear a rubber band on your wrist, and snap it when the thoughts begin."
   b. "Your thoughts are foolish and should be stopped."
   c. "Verbalizing the thoughts to someone else will help make them go away."
   d. "If you hurry through your ritualistic behaviors, you won't be bothered so much by them."

7. Ms. Martin has been hospitalized for treatment of dissociative identity disorder (multiple personality disorder). The nurse would most expect to find that Ms. Martin:

   a. Has a family history of dissociative identity disorder.
   b. Experienced childhood physical, emotional, or sexual abuse.
   c. Appears to hear voices at frequent intervals.
   d. Had a sudden onset of panic attacks.

8. Albert, a client with a diagnosis of chronic schizophrenia, throws a book across the room. "The voices told me to throw the

book," Albert tells the nurse. The nurse determines that Albert is experiencing which of the following?

a. Idea of reference
b. A command hallucination
c. A delusion of grandeur
d. Paranoia

9. In a client who is taking haloperidol (Haldol) for psychosis, which response indicates an acute dystonic reaction to the drug?

a. Restlessness and pacing
b. Drooling
c. A masklike expression
d. Muscle spasm

10. Conrad, who has been diagnosed with major depression, begins taking amitriptyline hydrochloride (Elavil), a tricyclic antidepressant. For which of the following common side effects does the nurse assess the client?

a. Dry mouth
b. Increased blood pressure
c. Diarrhea
d. Weight loss

11. Tonya Henson, who has been under treatment for depression, attempted suicide by taking her entire bottle of the tricyclic antidepressant imipramine hydrochloride (Tofranil). While she is being treated for the overdose, it will be critical to monitor her for which toxic effect?

a. Severe hypertension
b. Respiratory arrest
c. Acute renal failure
d. Cardiac arrhythmias

12. An appropriate nursing diagnosis to address potential side effects of lithium therapy for the treatment of bipolar disorder would be:

a. Constipation related to anticholinergic effects of the medication.
b. Altered oral mucous membranes related to dry mouth.
c. Sexual dysfunction related to decreased libido.
d. Fluid volume deficit related to polyuria.

13. Mr. Lin, who has moderate Alzheimer's disease, comes to the nurse's station and reports, "The man next door stole my razor." The most appropriate response by the nurse would be:

a. "Did you hide your razor again?"
b. "Mr. Hernandez didn't take your razor; you put it away."
c. "Let me help you look for your razor."
d. "I'll file a report, and we'll have it investigated."

14. Mr. Quinn is in the severe stage of Alzheimer's disease. When the nurse serves his lunch tray, he begins rearranging items on the tray and mumbling incoherently. The most effective nursing action would be to:

a. Interrupt Mr. Quinn's mumbling and ask, "How are you feeling right now?"
b. Recognize that Mr. Quinn is unable to feed himself, and assign an aide to feed him.
c. Prepare the items on the tray, hand him the fork, and observe whether he eats.
d. Say, "I see you're ready to eat now. May I help you cut your meat?"

15. Mrs. Finley will be caring for her husband, who has dementia, at home. In providing education and support to Mrs. Finley, the nurse should include which information?

a. Mrs. Finley needs to arrange some free time for her own personal activities.
b. Physical or chemical restraint will become necessary as wandering increases.
c. To promote reality orientation, Mrs. Finley needs to firmly correct her husband's inaccurate statements.
d. To prevent weight loss as the disease progresses, Mrs. Finley should increase her husband's portions at mealtimes.

16. The most useful physical assessment to evaluate the course of delirium is the:

a. Pulse.
b. Respiratory pattern.
c. Accuracy of perception.
d. Physical activity level.

17. According to psychologic theories, which of the following is associated with an increased risk of substance abuse?

   a. Parental overprotectiveness
   b. Assertiveness in early relationships
   c. Judgmental attitudes
   d. Compulsive adherence to rules

18. The nurse should consider amphetamine abuse in connection with which of the following assessment findings?

   a. Pupil constriction
   b. Sudden weight gain
   c. Irregular pulse
   d. Muscle atrophy

19. Mr. Pringle is being treated on the medical-surgical unit for alcohol-induced gastritis. When the nurse reminds him of the need to avoid alcohol, he states, "My job is very stressful. I just have a beer or 2 to unwind when I get home." Which response by the nurse would be most therapeutic?

   a. "I know what you mean. I often feel like having a drink when I get off duty."
   b. "How are you feeling about going back to work?"
   c. "It will be difficult to give up your drink after work. Have you thought about how you will handle that?"
   d. "Is the reduction of your stress for a short while worth the risk to your health?"

20. The nurse working with clients who have eating disorders will find which of the following features common to all these disorders?

   a. A biologic theory of causation
   b. Clients who have difficulty identifying and expressing needs
   c. Equal numbers of males and females
   d. Clients who struggle for perfection

21. The nurse is admitting Anna, age 14, who has a tentative diagnosis of anorexia nervosa. Which statement made by Anna to the nurse would indicate a need to reconsider the diagnosis?

   a. "I haven't had a period in a long time."
   b. "I'm afraid I'll gain weight and be fat."
   c. "I think I'm too thin to be pretty."
   d. "My nails break, and my hair falls out."

22. For a male client with a diagnosis of borderline personality disorder, the nurse develops a nursing diagnosis of ineffective individual coping related to anxiety as evidenced by angry outbursts. The best nursing intervention related to this diagnosis is to:

   a. Allow the client to determine his daily schedule.
   b. Encourage the client to express his anger.
   c. Provide the client with guidelines for acceptable behavior.
   d. Reduce stress for the client by avoiding confrontations.

23. A single mother asks the nurse, "Why does my 2-year-old son have temper tantrums?" The best response by the nurse would be to say:

   a. "He is expressing his independence."
   b. "Your discipline is inconsistent."
   c. "Boys need limits set by a man."
   d. "Your son's behavior indicates a developmental problem."

24. The nurse's ability to assess adequately a client's sexual functioning depends most on which of the following?

   a. The nurse's knowledge about human sexuality and sexual deviations
   b. The nurse's comfort in dealing with his/her own sexuality
   c. The client's attitude toward the nurse
   d. The institution's policy on sexual assessment

ANSWERS

1. **Correct answer is b.** Efficiency includes a therapeutic communication that is brief, clear, and has a focus. Flexibility is necessary to keep the process and feedback loop therapeutic. Appropriateness denotes the importance of the statement or feedback to the message delivered or received.

a. Honesty is important in building a therapeutic relationship and is necessary for facilitative communication, but it is not articulated in therapeutic communication. Redundancy is important in some learning activities, but it is not necessary for therapeutic communication. Rigidity is not therapeutic; it is counter to the fluidity that is needed.

c. Selectivity helps to focus, but it can also denote that a sent or received message could be inappropriately screened. Clarity is a component of efficiency. Receptivity is helpful, but it is not articulated as a concept that stands alone in therapeutic communication.

d. Engagement is an activity that may be a part of any interaction. Fluidity is a concept that denotes smoothness; therapeutic communication may not always be smooth. Therapeutic communication does not need to be eloquent. It is better to be simple.

2. **Correct answer is a.** Family therapists believe that a change in 1 individual affects the family as a whole; in addition, family illness is manifested in the problems exhibited by individual family members.

   b. Family therapy focuses on improving the health of all family members, not just the identified client. Symptoms of 1 family member are considered to be symptoms of family dysfunction rather than of individual illness.

   c. Family therapy is concerned with the relationships among family members, not with the function of individual members.

   d. Nurses work with families in various practice settings, but the practice of family therapy requires educational preparation at the master's level.

3. **Correct answer is d.** It is impossible to reassure the client until the nurse defines the exact nature of the client's concerns.

   a. This is a true statement, but it should not be used until the nurse determines exactly what has caused the client to worry.

b. In general, this is true, but the nurse needs to determine if the client is worried about safety or about some other aspect of ECT. As with any procedure requiring anesthesia, there is a small risk to the client.

c. Informed consent requires that clients have an understanding of the risks and benefits of procedures before giving consent. The nurse should identify and address any fears.

4. **Correct answer is d.** When asked to make a judgment about what to do with a stamped letter, a client with poor judgment and reasoning may choose to do nothing with the letter or to throw it away.

   a. This provides data about orientation to time.

   b. This provides data about orientation to reality.

   c. This provides data about mood.

5. **Correct answer is a.** The serial 7s test evaluates the client's ability to focus on a mental task.

   b. Reality orientation may be assessed by asking the client questions about time, place, or current events.

   c. Memory may be assessed by asking the client about recent and remote past.

   d. Speech may be assessed by listening to the client talk and by identifying factors such as whether speech is intelligible, fast, or slow.

6. **Correct answer is a.** Clients have found that self-controlled behavior modification such as snapping a rubber band can help interrupt obsessive thinking.

   b. The client already believes that obsessive thoughts are foolish, but the thoughts are not under voluntary control. Making the client feel foolish will increase the anxiety and the obsessive behavior.

   c. Once obsessive thoughts have been described, continued reiteration serves to reinforce rather than to reduce them.

   d. Hurrying increases a client's anxiety and may increase the need for the ritualistic behavior.

7. **Correct answer is b.** Dissociative identity disorder (multiple personality disorder) is almost always a response to abuse experienced in childhood. The child learns to use dissociation to avoid situations that produce extreme anxiety, and the pattern persists with any anxiety-provoking situation.

  a. Family history is not significant in this disorder.
  c. Hallucinations are not a part of this disorder.
  d. Panic attacks are not common with this disorder. The client deals with anxiety through dissociation.

8. **Correct answer is b.** Albert is experiencing an auditory hallucination that tells him to do a particular act.

  a. An idea of reference is a type of delusion in which the client falsely assumes that some trivial event has personal significance for him.
  c. Delusions of grandeur are false beliefs about power or self-importance.
  d. Paranoia is the false belief that others are plotting against oneself.

9. **Correct answer is d.** Dystonic reactions are spasms of voluntary muscles of the neck, back, jaws, limbs, and eyes. The nurse observes for this extrapyramidal side effect particularly during the first 5 days of haloperidol therapy. It requires immediate treatment with an intramuscular injection of diphenhydramine hydrochloride (Benadryl) or benztropine mesylate (Cogentin).

  a. Restlessness and pacing are signs of akathisia. This extrapyramidal side effect occurs in about 20% of clients taking antipsychotic medications.
  b and c. Drooling and masklike expression are signs of pseudoparkinsonism, another extrapyramidal side effect.

10. **Correct answer is a.** Dry mouth is one of the anticholinergic side effects common to tricyclic antidepressants.

  b. Tricyclics typically cause hypotension, not increases in blood pressure.

  c. Tricyclics typically cause constipation due to their anticholinergic effect.
  d. Weight gain, not weight loss, is typical of tricyclics.

11. **Correct answer is d.** At toxic levels, tricyclic antidepressants (TCAs) commonly induce dangerous arrhythmias.

  a. Orthostatic hypotension is a common side effect of TCAs. Hypertension would not be expected.
  b. Respiratory depression is not a major side effect of TCAs. Respiratory arrest is much more likely with CNS depressant drugs.
  c. TCAs are not highly nephrotoxic. Although acute renal failure may occur with any type of overdose, it is not common with tricyclics.

12. **Correct answer is d.** Polyuria often occurs in the first weeks of therapy and may result in fluid volume deficit if fluid intake is inadequate to replace lost fluid.

  a. Constipation may occur with tricyclic antidepressants (TCAs) but is unlikely with lithium. Diarrhea occurs with lithium toxicity.
  b. Dry mouth is not a common side effect of lithium. It does occur with TCAs and antipsychotic medications.
  c. Sexual dysfunction is not a common side effect of lithium. It is more likely to occur with TCAs or sedatives.

13. **Correct answer is c.** The nurse needs to respond to Mr. Lin's underlying need, which is to locate his razor. Offering to help look for the razor does not call attention to Mr. Lin's memory deficit, and it also does not support his inaccurate statement.

  a. Asking Mr. Lin if he hid his razor is a judgmental response that calls attention to the client's cognitive deficits and threatens his self-esteem.
  b. While presenting reality might be appropriate in other circumstances, it is likely to lead to an argument with the client who has Alzheimer's disease because the client is convinced of the truth of his statement and lacks insight into his deficits.

d. It is inappropriate to reinforce Mr. Lin's incorrect belief, which would be the effect of filing a report.

14. **Correct answer is d.** This provides guidance to Mr. Quinn about the task he is to perform without calling attention to his deficits. It also preserves his self-esteem by addressing him in an adult manner and soliciting his permission before giving help.

    a. In the severe stage of Alzheimer's disease, Mr. Quinn is incapable of insight into his responses. It is important to allow clients with a diagnosis of dementia to use denial as a defense mechanism, since their losses are devastating and irreversible, and their cognitive skills are insufficient to allow them to utilize more effective coping methods.
    b. Further assessment would be needed to determine whether Mr. Quinn cannot feed himself. His actions indicate only that he is unable to initiate the task without help. Imposing unneeded assistance infantilizes him unnecessarily.
    c. Mr. Quinn needs some direction for the task at hand. Giving him the fork will not accomplish this.

15. **Correct answer is a.** Altered family processes and caregiver role strain are major problems for families who provide home care for a family member who has dementia. Family members often fail to plan mental and physical rest for themselves. Since the care of individuals who have dementia is frustrating and often seems hopeless, the family needs to be encouraged to plan rest periods and vacations. By mentioning this information, the nurse "gives permission" for family self-care.

    b. Restraint of any kind should be avoided, since it increases the anxiety and behavior problems of the person who has dementia. Environmental modifications to make wandering safe or reduce motivation to wander need to be reviewed with the family.
    c. Mrs. Finley needs to be taught ways to avoid confronting her husband's misperceptions without reinforcing inaccurate information.

Engaging in arguments with him about his statements may precipitate physical violence.
d. As the disease progresses, wandering will increase, and it will be increasingly difficult to get Mr. Finley to remain at the table to complete a meal. Mrs. Finley should be advised to provide snacks, especially finger foods, with high nutritional value.

16. **Correct answer is a.** Autonomic signs often accompany delirium. When delirium is caused by metabolic abnormalities or substance withdrawal, monitoring pulse and blood pressure may be critical. The pulse is particularly useful because it provides a good indicator of the course of the delirium.

    b. Respiratory pattern is not a sensitive indicator of the autonomic changes that are the most likely physical correlates of delirium.
    c and **d.** Changes in perception and activity level do occur with delirium. They do not develop or resolve in a predictable way, however, so they do not provide a reliable measure of the progression of the delirium and recovery.

17. **Correct answer is c.** Judgmental attitudes that mask self-doubt are commonly associated with later substance abuse.

    a. A perception of one's parents as emotionally cold is more likely to be associated with increased risk of substance abuse.
    b. Insecurity and passivity, possibly masked by dominance in relationships, are common among persons at increased risk of substance abuse.
    d. Rebelliousness toward authority is more likely to be associated with substance abuse than is compliance.

18. **Correct answer is c.** Cardiac dysrhythmias often produce chest pain or irregular pulse in the individual who abuses amphetamines.

    a. Amphetamines cause pupil dilation.
    b. Amphetamine abuse may result in appetite suppression and increased metabolic rate, which usually lead to weight loss.
    d. Amphetamine intoxication may produce dyskinesias, dystonias, or muscle weakness. Muscle atrophy does not occur.

19. **Correct answer is c.** It is important for the nurse to be nonjudgmental and supportive. The nurse should first recognize that abstinence is difficult but then should direct the client's attention to healthier coping mechanisms.

a. This response reflects enabling by the nurse. By agreeing with the client's rationalization, the nurse encourages denial.

b. This response also reflects enabling by the nurse. By shifting to a different subject, the nurse helps the client avoid the topic of alcohol abuse.

d. This response is judgmental and suggests that the problem can be overcome by applying rational thinking and willpower.

20. **Correct answer is b.** Difficulty identifying and expressing needs has been noted in clients who have anorexia, bulimia, and obesity.

a. Biologic theories to explain eating disorders are not commonly accepted.

c. The majority of individuals with eating disorders are female (95%).

d. Although a struggle for perfection is common among clients who have anorexia, it is not consistently found among clients who have other eating disorders.

21. **Correct answer is c.** An outstanding characteristic of anorexia nervosa is distorted body image; even emaciated clients see themselves as fat.

a. Amenorrhea is a characteristic of malnutrition from any cause, including anorexia nervosa.

b. A pathologic fear of gaining weight is almost always present in anorexia nervosa.

d. Brittle hair and nails are characteristic of malnutrition and are frequently present in anorexia nervosa.

22. **Correct answer is c.** In clients with borderline personality disorder, structure and limits reduce anxiety and acting-out behavior.

a. Control issues are frequently problematic for the client with a diagnosis of borderline personality disorder. The most effective approach is for the treatment team to determine therapeutic activities.

b. Clients with a diagnosis of borderline personality disorder have excessive anger that is triggered by stress. Controlling the anger through stress reduction techniques would be more therapeutic than venting anger.

d. In the treatment setting, it is essential to confront negative behaviors to help the client grow and change.

23. **Correct answer is a.** Temper tantrums and negativism are normal states for a 2-year-old and represent the child's efforts to become more independent.

b. This statement indicates incorrectly that the mother is at fault for the occurrence of tantrums.

c. This statement indicates incorrectly that firmer discipline would eliminate the temper tantrums.

d. Because temper tantrums are normal for 2-year-olds, this statement is inappropriate. There are no data to indicate that the child has a developmental problem.

24. **Correct answer is b.** It is difficult for the nurse to create a climate in which a client is comfortable discussing sexual concerns if the nurse is not comfortable with his/her own feelings and sexuality.

a. Knowledge is helpful, but the nurse's attitude is of primary importance.

c. The client may need education to recognize the nurse as a possible source of assistance for sexual concerns, but this can be accomplished once the nurse is comfortable with his/her own sexuality.

d. The nurse should be aware of any relevant policies, but the greatest obstacle to adequate assessment is the nurse's own anxiety.